Foodborne disease
a focus for health education

◆◆◆

World Health Organization
Geneva
2000

WHO Library Cataloguing-in-Publication Data

Food-borne disease : a focus for health education.

1.Food hygiene   2.Health education   3.Food contamination   4.Food handling   5.Disease transmission − prevention and control   6.Enterobacteriaceae infections − prevention and control   7.Consumer participation

ISBN 92 4 156196 3   (NLM classification: WA 701)

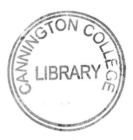

Designed in New Zealand
Typeset in Hong Kong
Printed in Malta
98/12231−minimum graphics/Best-set/Interprint−7000

Contents

Preface

WHO has recognized the importance of education of food handlers and consumers for a number of years. In 1983, the Joint FAO/WHO Expert Committee on Food Safety, which discussed the role of food safety in health and development (Geneva, 1983), identified public education and community participation as essential pillars of strategies for improving food safety and for intervening to prevent foodborne disease. As a follow-up to this Expert Committee, a consultation on health education in food safety in 1987 gave further guidance in this regard. Since then numerous efforts have been made to promote health education in food safety, and several publications and educational materials have been developed for this purpose.

The present book is intend to highlight the public health aspects of food safety. It is an invitation to all who are concerned with food safety and public health education to make every effort to further educate consumers and train food handlers. It tries to capture the concept developed at the WHO consultation on health education in food safety, while at the same time reflecting the extensive experience of WHO's programme on food safety in terms of prevailing fallacies and the need for guidance.

At the time when the plans for this book were first laid some years ago, public health authorities were paying little attention to food safety and even less to health education in food safety. Today there is greater awareness and recognition of the importance of food safety for public health and development in some countries. This may be partly due to WHO's advocacy, but the subject has also received publicity as a result of some important events.

The large-scale outbreak of cholera in Peru and other Latin American countries in the early 1990s was a turning point in that it drew the attention of public health authorities to the link between food and cholera—a link that had previously been overlooked. The epidemic had devastating effects on the health and economy of several countries.

Within the context of the General Agreement on Tariffs and Trade (GATT), the Uruguay Round of Multilateral Trade Negotiations was successfully concluded in April 1994, resulting in liberalization of the food trade. According to the Agreement on the Application of Sanitary and Phytosanitary Measures the work of Codex Alimentarius Commission (through the establishment of standards, guidelines and recommendations) has been recognized as the reference for national food safety requirements. This implies that countries that are involved in international trade and that are members of the World Trade Organization can no longer reject foodstuffs which meet Codex standards, recommendations or guidelines without providing justification. Although these developments have concerned principally the regulatory approach to food safety and the need for countries to update their food control systems, they have nevertheless sparked off a debate regarding the responsibilities of consumers and food handlers in food safety and the need for definition of the degree of safety that should be expected from producers and processors.

Other controversial issues, such as the problem of bovine spongiform encephalopathy (BSE) and the use of hormones in food production, have also called into question modern methods of food production and the measures taken to ensure food safety. In addition, the problem of dioxin in animal feed has increased consumer concern.

Perhaps the most important factor in increasing the concern of public health authorities in some countries (mainly industrialized) has been the increasing incidence of foodborne illnesses and a series of outbreaks with fatal or severe health consequences. Some outbreaks were of massive proportions, affecting hundreds of thousands of people; others caused consternation and apprehension because of their severity or the number of deaths that resulted as well as their new epidemiological features. Weaknesses in investigation and surveillance systems for foodborne diseases in developing countries have meant that alarming figures or news about such outbreaks have been relatively scarce, but countries have been alerted worldwide to potential problems looming in the area of food safety and the potential increase and spread of foodborne illnesses.

The climate of concern among food control and public health authorities, as well as industries and consumers, has been an impetus for many governments to take a fresh look at their food safety programmes and to pay greater attention to information, education and training of food handlers. Nevertheless, the subject is far from receiving the attention that it deserves and in most countries the issue of food safety, and in particular health education in food safety, is frequently overlooked or receives low priority in public health programmes.

Even in countries where the authorities are conscious of the problem, very few have taken the step from recognition to action by developing a comprehensive, systematic and continuous programme of health education based on modern approaches to food safety. Several of the reviewers of this book requested examples of success stories regarding health education in food safety and failure to do so is an indication of the small amount of work that has been done in this area. Unfortunately, even where educational activities in food safety have been carried out, the activities have often not been properly coordinated with those primarily concerned, or the programme has lacked proper planning or evaluation that would have enabled improvements and adjustments to be made. Many attempts have also been based on traditional or outdated approaches to hygiene education, with the result that some of these activities have done more harm than good.

Admittedly the situation has changed greatly over the last few years, and today in some countries there is a greater awareness among consumers. However, in many instances this change has been a consequence of negative publicity in the media, leading to a feeling of insecurity among consumers rather than to a sustained information and education campaign about consumer roles and responsibilities. While this book was in preparation new data became available that could not be included but that clearly supported the book's message. Therefore, the need to produce this book has persisted, and it is hoped that it will achieve its objectives of raising awareness of the need for health education in food safety and of prompting actions. Even if it succeeds only in stimulating scientific debate and research, it will have accomplished a great deal in enhancing the know-how of the scientific community and shaping its views in this important area.

Finally, the attention of the reader is drawn to the sad story of Dr Ignaz Semmelweiss (1818–1865) and the lesson that we should learn from it. For years, thousands of women lost their lives simply because of the unwillingness of his peers to recognize the importance of his discovery and to follow his recommendations with regard to washing their hands in order to prevent perinatal infections. It is strongly hoped that this book can bring a change in health education in food safety and that the recommendations in it will be duly considered by the relevant authorities.

Acknowledgements

This publication has been prepared by Dr Yasmine Motarjemi, Scientist, Food Safety programme, WHO, with contributions from Dr Akbar Moarefi, former Chief, WHO Health Education programme, and Mr Mike Jacob, consultant in food safety and food law, United Kingdom. The book is the result of collaboration between WHO's Food Safety and Health Education and Health Promotion programmes.

The following persons reviewed the book and provided valuable comments and suggestions:

Professor M. Abdussalam, Pakistan and Germany

Ms Akosua Asante, Food Safety, WHO, Geneva, Switzerland

Dr Michele Beaudry, UNICEF, New York, USA

Dr John S. Crowther, UNILEVER Research, Bedford, England (on behalf of the Industry Council for Development)

Professor Michael P. Doyle, University of Georgia, USA (on behalf of International Life Sciences Institute, Washington, DC, USA)

Professor Layi Erinosho, Ogun State University, Nigeria

Dr Jack Theodore Jones, Division of Health Promotion, Education and Communication, WHO, Geneva, Switzerland

Mrs Joanna Koch, Convener of the NGO Working Group on Nutrition, Kilchberg, Switzerland

Professor Rolf Korte, Deutsche Gesellschaft für Technische Zusammenarbeit (GTZ), Eschborn, Germany

Dr Raj K. Malik, New Delhi, India

Professor Silvia C. Michanie, Buenos Aires, Argentina

Dr Serve Notermans, WHO Collaborating Centre for Microbiological Aspects of Food Safety, Bilthoven, Netherlands

Dr Fernando Quevedo, Lima, Peru

Dr Jocelyne Rocourt, Pasteur Institute, Paris, France

Group Captain Roger A. Smith, Secretary, Royal Institute of Public Health and Hygiene, London, England

Dr Eghbal Taheri, Ministry of Health and Medical Education, Teheran, Islamic Republic of Iran

Mr Robert Tanner, National Sanitation Foundation International, Brussels, Belgium

Mrs Susan Van der Vynckt, UNESCO, Paris, France

The following WHO programmes assisted in revising the text: Nutrition, Rural Environmental Health, Child Health and Development.

WHO would like also to express its appreciation to the International Life Sciences Institute (ILSI) for its financial support towards the preparation of this book.

Introduction

Foodborne diseases are a widespread public health problem and a significant cause of reduced economic productivity. Each year throughout the world, millions of people, particularly infants and children, suffer and die from foodborne diseases (1). While the role of food producers and processors in ensuring food safety should not be underestimated, many cases of foodborne illnesses, if not most, could be prevented—and many lives saved—if food handlers were better educated and trained in safe food-handling and consumers were better advised in the choice of their food.[1]

The importance of food safety, and particularly the need for education about it, has been highlighted at many international meetings. The WHO/UNICEF International Conference on Primary Health Care (Alma-Ata, 1978) proclaimed that "education concerning prevailing health problems and the methods of preventing and controlling them" is an essential element of primary health care. Promotion of the food supply and proper nutrition were considered to be other essential components (2). The importance of the subject was reiterated at the World Summit for Children (New York, 1990), the United Nations Conference on Environment and Health (Rio de Janeiro, 1992) and the International Conference on Nutrition (Rome, 1992). In its Plan of Action, the Rome conference made the recommendation to "support consumer education to contribute to an educated and knowledgeable public, safe practices in the home, community participation and active consumer associations" (1).

In response to this call for the promotion of health education, including food safety, the Forty-second World Health Assembly passed a resolution (WHA42.44) in 1989 requesting WHO to support Member States in strengthening national capabilities in all aspects of health promotion, public information and education for health. It also requested that particular attention be paid to the development of new and effective methodologies and strategies. Later, the Forty-sixth World Health Assembly passed a resolution (WHA46.7) urging Member States to reduce foodborne diseases by the year 2000 and to remedy poor hygiene.

Independently of these developments, the General Assembly of the United Nations adopted on 9 April 1985 guidelines for consumer protection in which

---

[1] The term "food" is taken here to include drinking-water and water used in food preparation. In certain circumstances water is referred to as a separate entity.

it encouraged countries, and particularly developing countries, to develop consumer education programmes. The protection of consumers from hazards to their health and safety, the access of consumers to adequate information to enable them to make informed choices according to their wishes and needs, and consumer education are principles of these guidelines (*3*).

In spite of this recognition, food safety, and in particular the education of consumers and food handlers in food safety, has often been given very low priority in national health programmes. Further, the significance of food safety has often not been recognized in programmes for the prevention of diarrhoea. In a review of 67 articles that described and evaluated health education programmes in developing countries, none of the studies was designed to educate consumers/food handlers in food safety (*4*). Although the importance of food safety is being increasingly recognized, neglect of this subject in the past has perpetuated the high prevalence of diarrhoeal diseases. Many hygiene education programmes for the prevention of diarrhoeal diseases have not been very effective, since issues of food safety have not been considered.

One of the factors contributing to the scant attention to this subject is perhaps the insufficient awareness of health policy-makers and medical and health personnel of the health consequences of food contamination and the links between many diseases and food. The purpose of this book is therefore to:

— raise the awareness of health policy-makers of the importance of foodborne diseases for public health and outline the scope of food safety problems;

— highlight the importance of the education of food handlers and consumers for the prevention of foodborne illnesses;

— describe approaches used to select health education messages and key behaviours that need to be changed or reinforced;

— suggest possible partners or channels for implementation and communication, drawing on past experiences and initiatives or existing materials as examples of how objectives can be achieved.

The term "education" (in the context of the expression *health education in food safety*) is used in this book in its broadest sense and includes all types of activities, from communication and information to training, which enable the target audience to acquire the know-how and skills necessary to understand and manage food safety hazards. Strictly speaking, there is a distinction between training and education. Training is a process by which one is enabled to acquire a skill, while education—particularly health education—aims at influencing the way of life and empowering people to make a reasonable and informed choice without imposing preconceived values. The views expressed in the educational interventions do not necessarily represent the views of WHO. The initiatives and educational material presented in this book are given only as examples of efforts that have already been made.

The book emphasizes microbial and parasitic foodborne illnesses as these account for most episodes of acute foodborne disease and because education can help consumers and food handlers to play a greater role in their prevention. The term "food handlers" is taken to mean all people who handle, prepare or serve food, be they domestic food handlers (preparing family food) or professional food handlers such as those working in food service or catering establishments (cooks, waiters), retail stores, supermarkets, cottage industries or small businesses (e.g. bakeries) or street food vendors. Depending on their tasks, other professionals such as nurses and flight attendants may also be food handlers. Food handlers working in medium and large industries require education and training in food safety. However, this book focuses on operations where regulatory agencies have little or no power to control the safety of prepared food and where the type of food prepared often changes.

- Chapter 1 describes the extent of the problem of foodborne diseases. It outlines the nature of foodborne diseases, trends, economic implications, emerging pathogens and factors that affect prevalence. By citing examples, the chapter demonstrates the formidable task that is before the health sector.

- Chapter 2 gives 10 reasons why health education in food safety is both necessary and effective. It calls for the systematic education and training of professional food handlers, and for increased consumer information.

- Chapter 3 explains the complexity of behaviours that have an influence on food safety and describes approaches that have been used in selecting behaviours as the focus for change. Particular emphasis is given to the Hazard Analysis Critical Control Point (HACCP) system, which is a modern approach to food safety assurance that also has applications for health education about food safety.

- Chapter 4 suggests strategies and partners for educational programmes and draws on initiatives from different countries as examples.

- Chapter 5 gives guidance in implementing educational programmes and the infrastructure needed for the design and planning of such programmes, without extending to behavioural sciences and educational methods, for which references to appropriate publications are provided (5–8).

- Following the conclusion, Annex 1 contains a series of tables on the characteristics, transmission and prevention of foodborne illnesses, while Annex 2 describes the issue of risk communication as an element of health education.

The information and examples in this book have been drawn from a wide variety of sources around the world. However, much of the work in the area of health education for food safety has taken place in developed countries. Examples from these countries may predominate in some parts of the book because of the limited extent of this kind of activity elsewhere.

A number of other WHO books deal with related topics. *Education for health* (*9*) explains methods of education, *Safe food-handling* (*10*) is an application of food safety to food and catering establishments, and *Basic food safety for health workers* is a resource book for health workers (*11*).

The primary target audiences of this book are health policy-makers, the managers of food safety and health education programmes in both the public and private sectors, and consumer bodies. The book is also intended for those working in cooperation and development agencies, national and international organizations, academic institutions, nongovernmental organizations and all who have responsibility for public health protection and promotion.

References

1. FAO/WHO. *International Conference on Nutrition. World Declaration and Plan of Action for Nutrition, Rome, December 1992.* Geneva, World Health Organization, 1992 (unpublished document ICN/92/2; available on request from Nutrition, World Health Organization, 1211 Geneva 27, Switzerland).

2. *Primary health care. Report of the International Conference on Primary Health Care, Alma-Ata, USSR, 6–12 September 1978.* Geneva, World Health Organization, 1978.

3. *Guidelines for consumer protection.* New York, United Nations, 1986.

4. Loevinsohn BP. Health education interventions in developing countries: a methodological review of published articles. *International journal of epidemiology*, 1990, 19(4):788–794.

5. Green LW, Kreuter M. *Health promotion planning: an educational and environmental approach.* Mountain View, CA, Mayfield Publishing Company, 1991.

6. Arnhold W et al. *Healthy eating for young people in Europe: nutrition education in health promoting schools* (draft). Kiel, Ministry of Education of Schleswig-Holstein, 1995.

7. *Facts for life. Lessons from experience.* New York, United Nations Children's Fund, 1996.

8. Srinivasan L. *Tools for community participation: a manual for training trainers in participatory technique.* New York, United Nations Development Programme, 1990.

9. *Education for health: a manual on health education in primary health care.* Geneva, World Health Organization, 1988.

10. *Safe food handling. A training guide for managers of food service establishments.* Geneva, World Health Organization, 1989.

11. *Basic food safety for health workers.* Geneva, World Health Organization, 1999 (unpublished document WHO/SDE/PHE/99.1; available on request from Food Safety, World Health Organization, 1211 Geneva 27, Switzerland).

CHAPTER 1

Foodborne diseases: a global health and economic problem

Foodborne diseases, usually either infectious or toxic in nature, are caused by agents that enter the body through the ingestion of contaminated food. These diseases are sometimes inaccurately referred to as "food poisoning". They include a range of diseases of chemical and biological origin, including cholera and diarrhoeal diseases, as well as a number of parasitic diseases.

Foodborne diseases represent one of the most widespread and overwhelming public health problems of the modern world. They take a heavy toll of human life and cause a great deal of suffering, particularly among infants, children, the elderly and persons who are immunocompromised. The magnitude and consequences of foodborne diseases are often underestimated by public health authorities. Only in recent years, as a consequence of several life-threatening foodborne disease outbreaks (e.g. outbreaks of enterohaemorrhagic *Escherichia coli* infection, listeriosis, salmonellosis and cholera), has awareness increased in some countries of the significance of these diseases for public health. Nevertheless, resources for the prevention of foodborne diseases are lacking. Regrettably, the countries that bear the biggest burden of the problem are also the ones that have the fewest resources to prevent it. Due to the broadness of the subject, the lack of information in some parts of the world and the fragmentary nature of it in others, it is not possible to review or compare data from different countries. Thus, this chapter attempts to give an insight into the scope, magnitude, nature, and health and economic consequences of foodborne diseases and the factors that affect their prevalence. Some of the examples provided here are selected especially to illustrate faulty practices and to show the need for health education in food safety. Although this chapter deals separately with the problems of developing and industrialized countries, it should be realized that diseases have no boundaries and most of them occur worldwide, regardless of region or stage of development.

Magnitude and nature of foodborne diseases

Developing countries

Developing countries are affected by a wide range of foodborne diseases. Cholera, campylobacteriosis, *E. coli* gastroenteritis, salmonellosis, shigellosis, typhoid and paratyphoid fevers, brucellosis, amoebiasis and poliomyelitis are only a few examples (*1*). With poor or non-existent reporting systems in most countries, reliable statistics on these diseases are not available and their magnitude is therefore difficult to estimate. The gravity of the situation can, however, be appreciated in view of the high prevalence of diarrhoeal diseases in infants and children. Each year some 1500 million episodes of diarrhoea occur in children under the age of five, and over 3 million children die as a direct result. Indirectly, many millions more die from the combined effects of diarrhoea and malnutrition (2). It was previously thought that contaminated water supplies were the main source of pathogens causing diarrhoea, but it is now recognized that food plays an equally important role. It is estimated that up to 70% of cases of diarrhoeal disease may be caused by contaminated food (3, 4). This includes drinking-water and water used for food preparation. It should be noted that the roles of water and food in transmission of diarrhoeal diseases cannot be dissociated as water is both an ingredient of food and drink and is also used for washing hands, food and utensils. Where water is contaminated and good hygienic practice is lacking, it is likely that food is also contaminated.

Pathogens which have been identified as the cause of diarrhoeal diseases include bacteria such as pathogenic *E. coli*, *Shigella* spp., *Salmonella* spp., *Vibrio cholerae* O1 and *Campylobacter jejuni*; protozoa such as *Giardia lamblia*, *Entamoeba histolytica*, *Cryptosporidium* spp; and also enteric viruses such as rotavirus (5). Infections due to pathogenic strains of *E. coli* are probably the commonest cause of diarrhoea in developing countries. They are responsible for up to 25% of diarrhoeal disease in infants and children and have been specifically associated with complementary foods[1] (3, 5). The frequent contamination of foods with *E. coli* and pathogens of faecal origin, as reported in the literature, signifies the contamination of food with faecal matter. Consequently, any pathogen known to be transmitted by the so-called faecal–oral route (e.g. rotavirus) can be transmitted through food (6). The role of food in the faecal–oral transmission of pathogens is shown in Fig. 1. Table 1 shows the pathogens that are frequently identified in children with acute diarrhoea seen at treatment centres in developing countries (5).

The contamination of complementary foods used in poor populations in developing countries is a daunting problem. Its role in diarrhoeal diseases and malnutrition has often been overlooked in the past. Numerous studies have shown that, in some populations, complementary foods are highly contaminated, that the level of contamination increases during the warm season and that complementary foods may often be more contaminated than adult foods (3).

---

[1] The period during which foods or liquids are provided along with breast milk is considered the period of complementary feeding. Any non-breast milk foods given to young children during the period of complementary feeding are defined as complementary foods. Sometimes the term "weaning" is used. As this term may imply a complete cessation of breast-feeding, it should not be used.

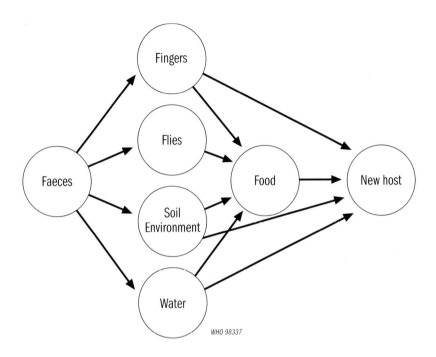

WHO 98337

Fig. 1. Role of food in the faecal–oral transmission of pathogens (Source: adapted from *6*)

Cholera is a serious problem in developing countries because of its health and socioeconomic consequences. In 1991, it spread to Latin America where some 595 000 people became infected and 19 295 died (*7*). In 1997, 65 countries, mainly in Africa, Asia and Latin America, were affected; over 147 000 cases of the disease were officially reported and 6274 people died. As for other diarrhoeal diseases, it was formerly believed that water was the vehicle for transmission of cholera. However, an increasing number of epidemiological studies have shown that food is an equally important route of transmission (*8, 9*). Table 2 (*10–43*) lists some examples of foodborne outbreaks of cholera. In Latin America, raw or undercooked seafood and beverages containing ice were important vehicles

Table 1. Pathogens that are frequently identified in children with acute diarrhoea seen at treatment centres in developing countries (Source: 5)

Pathogen	Percentage
Rotavirus	15-25
Escherichia coli	
– enterotoxigenic	10-20
– enteropathogenic	1-5
Shigella spp.	5-15
Campylobacter jejuni	10-15
Vibrio cholerae 01	5-10
Salmonella (non-typhi)	1-5
Cryptosporidium spp.	5-15

Table 2. Examples of foodborne outbreaks of cholera reported in the literature (Source: *8, 9*)

Year	Place	Food	No. of cases	Reference
1962	Philippines	Raw shrimp	–	*10*
1963	Hong Kong	Cold cooked meat	5	*11*
1970	Israel	Raw vegetables	258	*12*
1972	Australia	Mixed hors d'oeuvre	25	*13*
1973	Italy	Raw mussels, clams	278	*14*
1974	Portugal	Bottled mineral water	136	*15*
1974	Portugal	Seafood	2467	*16*
1974–1986	Guam	Raw seafoods	19–46	*17*
1977	Gilbert Islands	Raw and salted fish and clams	572	*18*
1978	Singapore	Steamed prawn, chicken, rice	12	*19*
1978	USA	Crabs	11	*20*
1978	Bahrain	Bottle-feeding of infants	42	*21*
1978	Japan	Rock lobster	18	*22*
1979	Spain	Raw fish	267	*23*
1981	USA	Cooked rice	15	*24*
1982	Micronesia (Federated States of)	Shellfish/leftover rice	509	*25*
1982	Singapore	Cooked squids	22	*26*
1984	India	Ice candies	46	*27*
1984	Mali	Millet gruel	1793	*28*
1986	Guinea	Peanut sauce/cooked rice	35	*29*
1986	USA	Crabs/shrimp	18	*30*
1986	USA	Raw oysters	2	*31*
1987	Thailand	Raw pork	130	*32*
1988	Thailand	Raw beef	52	*33*
1989	Philippines	Street food	–	*34*
1991	USA	Imported crabs	4	*35*
1991	Ecuador	Seafood	–	*36*
1991	USA	Imported frozen coconut milk	3	*37*
1991	Japan	Imported clams	21	*38*
1993	Guatemala	Leftover rice	26	*39*
1994	USA	Imported food (palm fruit)	2	*40*
1994	Thailand	Yellow rice	6	*41*
1994	El Salvador	Street food	541	*42*
1994	Hong Kong	Seafood	12	*43*

of transmission. In Latin America, as elsewhere, street food vendors have played an important role in the transmission of foodborne cases of cholera. Some studies have demonstrated that foods play an even greater role than water in causing this infection; many foods support the growth of *V. cholerae* to disease-causing levels and may also protect the microorganism from gastric acidity (*44*). The minimum infective dose of *V. cholerae* is high (10^6–10^8) and this is more easily reached in food subject to time–temperature abuse.[1] The alkalinity of certain foods may neutralize gastric acidity, with the result that *V. cholerae* is more likely to survive. It should, however, be remembered that water remains an important source of food contamination.

Refugee camps have frequently been traps for cholera and other epidemic diarrhoeal diseases. During 1992, in the Lisungwi camp that housed 60 000 refugees from Mozambique, 772 cases of abdominal cramps and bloody diarrhoea were documented. The major factor contributing to illness was consumption of cooked food bought at the market (*45*). Documented reports of other types of foodborne illness in refugee camps are not frequent, but this may be due to the fact that foodborne disease problems are often overshadowed by epidemic diarrhoeal diseases such as cholera and shigellosis and by other health and logistic problems. An outbreak of mass intoxication was reported in a camp for refugee children in Goma in the Democratic Republic of the Congo (formerly Zaire) in 1994 (*46*).

Other foodborne pathogens that are common in both developing and industrialized countries are *Bacillus cereus*, *Staphylococcus aureus* and *Clostridium perfringens*. These cause diseases that are frequently accompanied by diarrhoea. The incidence of infections/intoxications caused by these pathogens is probably very high all over the world; however, as the diseases are often self-limiting they receive little attention in public health services. They are principally associated with the time–temperature abuse of food during preparation and storage. In several Latin American countries (such as Brazil, Cuba and Venezuela), intoxications due to *Staphylococcus aureus* were the leading cause of foodborne disease outbreaks in the 1980s (*47, 48*).

Intoxications due to *Clostridium botulinum*, although rather rare, may be very severe and are sometimes deadly. Botulinum is one of the most powerful toxins known. Although industrially manufactured food has also been implicated in outbreaks of botulism, most cases occur as a result of faulty preservation or processing of food in homes. In China from 1958 to 1989, there were 745 reported outbreaks of botulism involving 2861 cases and 421 deaths. Over 62% of the cases were caused by home-made fermented bean products stored in

---

[1] Time–temperature abuse refers to situations where food has not been cooked for long enough or at a sufficiently high temperature to reduce contaminants to safe levels, or food has been stored for a time or at a temperature that permits bacteria to proliferate.

earthenware jars and other containers (*49*). It should be noted that botulism is not exclusive to developing countries and that it occurs all over the world. Foods frequently implicated in botulism in the USA (excluding Alaska) and southern Europe are home-preserved vegetables. In the native population of Alaska, where the incidence of botulism is particularly high, the foods primarily involved are fermented or putrefied fish and sea mammals. In France, Germany, Italy and Poland the main food involved has been meat such as home-cured ham (*50–52*).

Infections due to parasites are a great cause of concern, in terms of both magnitude and health consequences. Amoebiasis caused by *Entamoeba histolytica* is responsible for up to 100 000 deaths per year, which means that it ranks second only to malaria in mortality due to protozoan parasites (*53*). Other examples are helminthic infections due to *Trichinella spiralis*, *Taenia saginata* and *Taenia solium* which are acquired through the consumption of raw or uncooked meat. These parasites present an important public health problem in countries where there is a habit of consuming raw or underprocessed meat and where uninspected slaughtering of animals takes place. Outbreaks of trichinellosis are reported from Europe, Latin America and south-east Asia in connection with the consumption of raw or undercooked cured fermented pork or game meat (salami). An outbreak of trichinellosis associated with the ingestion of meat from a wild boar has been reported from Ethiopia, where 20 of the 30 persons who consumed the meat were affected (*54*). *Trichinella spiralis* may persist for months in cured uncooked products. Ascariasis, transmitted via contaminated vegetables and other means, is one of the most common parasitic infections that is estimated to affect over 1000 million people (*55*).

Trematodes such as *Clonorchis* spp., *Fasciola* spp., *Opisthorchis* spp. and *Paragonimus* spp. infect some 40 million people, particularly in Africa, Asia and Latin America. More than 10% of the world's population is at risk of becoming infected by these parasites, which are transmitted through the consumption of raw or inadequately processed freshwater fish, shellfish or aquatic plants (*56*).

Among viral infections, hepatitis A and rotavirus infection are of worldwide importance. Annually, some 10–50 people per 100 000 are affected by hepatitis A (*57*). Food handlers are a major source of contamination of food and many cases of hepatitis A are known to be associated with restaurants. The hepatitis A virus (HAV) may remain viable for several days or longer in contaminated food. HAV in fresh or salt water can also be concentrated in molluscs, making them also an important source of infection in humans (*58*). In 1988, a major epidemic of hepatitis A in China affected some 300 000 people and killed nine persons. The outbreak was traced to the consumption of contaminated clams (*59–61*). In several industrialized countries, bivalve molluscs—particularly raw oysters—have been implicated in outbreaks of hepatitis A. Hepatitis E, transmitted by the faecal–oral route, occurs widely in Africa, Asia and Latin

America. Although few foodborne outbreaks have been documented, waterborne outbreaks are common in developing countries (*62*).

Foodborne disease outbreaks due to small round-structured viruses (SRSV) are probably common worldwide, although statistical data are not available except in a few industrialized countries. In the United Kingdom SRSV account for 6% of foodborne disease outbreaks (*63, 64*). Bivalve molluscs such as oysters, cockles and mussels are the major food vehicles. Other types of food can also be contaminated with SRSV during preparation. Data from the United Kingdom show that 20–25% of all SRSV-positive outbreaks are related to food and that the implicated food was prepared by a food handler who was suffering from an illness with typical symptoms prior to the outbreak or had laboratory evidence of SRSV infection. Studies have shown that the route of transmission is not solely faecal contamination but also includes vomit (*64, 65*). It has been suggested that vomiting could liberate over 20 million virus particles. In addition to gross contamination, vomit can produce aerosols which in turn can contaminate food and work surfaces (*65*).

Among other foodborne hazards, there are naturally occurring toxins, and plant and marine biotoxins, that cause severe intoxications in both developing and industrialized countries. Ciguatera is one of the most common types of fish poisoning. It is associated with the consumption of certain tropical and subtropical fish—mainly predatory coral fish consuming other coral fish. There are an estimated 50 000 cases worldwide each year (*66*). During the last two decades several thousand cases of ciguatera have been reported from tropical and subtropical areas such as the Caribbean and Pacific (*1*). Studies in the Virgin Islands indicate an estimated annual incidence of 7.3–30 intoxications per 1000 persons (*67*). In addition to reef fish, shark has also been implicated in episodes of ciguatera–like intoxication. In 1993, some 200 persons were intoxicated in Madagascar following ingestion of shark, with an overall fatality rate of 30% (*68*).

Various types of shellfish poisoning are also reported from around the world. The toxins causing shellfish poisoning are produced by various species of dinoflagellates which, under certain conditions of light, temperature, salinity and nutrient supply, may multiply and form dense blooms. Until 1970, shellfish poisoning was reported mainly from Europe and North America. During recent decades, areas affected by these toxic blooms have increased and poisoning is appearing in regions of the world where it has not been known before (*69*). In 1980 the first outbreak of paralytic shellfish poisoning (PSP) occurred in Argentina due the blooming of *Alexandrium tamarense*. The toxic area has now expanded to cover nearly all of the Argentine coastal ecosystem. Similar problems are reported from Chile where, during a three-month period from October to December 1992, 295 people in Magellan were afflicted with PSP, with 18 fatalities. The fatality rate of 2–14% has been observed in regions of the world where the population has never before encountered the disease (*69*).

Mycotoxins are of major concern in developing countries as they may cause severe acute as well as chronic health effects. Aflatoxin is the best known and most important mycotoxin from the public health point of view. Fatal outbreaks of aflatoxicosis, caused by inadequate post-harvest handling of foods, have been reported from several countries with hot and humid climates, such as India and Malaysia (*70, 71*). Besides acute intoxications, mycotoxins are capable of having carcinogenic, mutagenic and teratogenic effects. Epidemiological studies show a strong correlation between the high incidence of liver cancer in some African and south-east Asian countries (i.e. 12–13 per 100000 annually) and exposure to aflatoxin. Certain studies suggest that aflatoxin and hepatitis B are co-carcinogens and the probability of liver cancer is higher in areas where both aflatoxin and hepatitis B are prevalent (*72*). Aflatoxin is found mostly in oilseeds (e.g. peanuts), cereals, tree nuts and some fruits such as figs. Ochratoxin A, patulin and fumonisin are three other mycotoxins of concern. Besides environmental conditions, the type of food and its post-harvest handling play an important role in the growth of moulds and the elaboration of mycotoxin (*73, 74*).

Intoxication due to other naturally occurring toxins, accidental consumption of pesticides, and adulteration are also common in developing countries. A major outbreak caused by pyrrolizidine alkaloids occurred in Tajikistan in 1992 when at least 3906 persons were intoxicated, resulting in severe liver injury and veno-occlusive disease. Over 2580 were aged under 15 years, and 52 died. The outbreak was due to the consumption of bread made with wheat mixed with seeds of *Heliotropium ellipticium* and *Trichodesma* (*75*).

Pesticide intoxications may also occur occasionally as a result of misuse, unsafe packaging, mislabelling or leakage of pesticide during storage or transport. In rural areas, accidental intoxication due to the use in food of insecticides mistaken for salt, sugar or flour is not uncommon. In Thailand, between 1981 and 1987, insecticides accounted for 27.4–58.4% of outbreaks (*76, 77*). Consumption of seeds treated with fungicides and intended for planting, or of contaminated fish caught in rice ponds, has also been a source of major intoxications. One of the most catastrophic outbreaks of methyl mercury poisoning ever recorded took place in Iraq during the winter of 1971–1972. More than 6000 persons were admitted to hospital and many more had mild symptoms. The cause of the outbreak was consumption of wheat treated with methyl mercury fungicide (*78*). A similar mass intoxication due to consumption of bread made with treated seed grain occurred in south-eastern Turkey where 3000–4000 people were affected, with a fatality rate of 10% (*79*).

While there is generally a lack of data from developing countries, data from developed countries on foods imported from developing countries indicate that these foods may contain high levels of pesticide residues. Information on organochlorine pesticide residues in the breast milk of women in developing countries is further evidence of significant cumulative exposure to these chemicals (*80, 81*).

Industrialized countries

Improvements in standards of personal hygiene, the development of basic sanitation, safe water supplies, effective vaccination programmes, food control infrastructure, and the increasing application of technologies such as pasteurization have either eradicated or considerably reduced many foodborne diseases (e.g. poliomyelitis, brucellosis, cholera, typhoid and paratyphoid fevers, and milkborne salmonellosis) in industrialized countries. Nevertheless, foodborne diseases remain a widespread public health problem in these countries. In 1990, an average of 120 cases per 100 000 were reported from 11 countries in Europe (*82*). The actual incidence is probably much higher. Surveys in New Zealand, Europe and North America suggest that each year up to 10% of the population may suffer from a foodborne disease (Table 3) (*83–95*). The estimated annual incidence of foodborne diseases in the USA has been estimated to be as high as 30–33 million, with about 9000 deaths per year (*87, 94, 95*). In 1995, salmonellosis, hepatitis A and shigellosis (all potentially foodborne) were among the 10 most frequently reported nationally notifiable infectious diseases. In children under the age of 5 years incidence rates of 61.8 for salmonellosis and 46.3 for shigellosis per 100 000 were reported (*96*). A survey in Sweden has indicated that annually some 79 persons per 1000 in the age group 16–74 suffer from a foodborne disease (*83*). Similarly, a sentinel study has shown that annually a total of 4.5 million cases of acute gastroenteritis occur in the Netherlands (population 15 million). It is estimated that about one-third of these cases, i.e. 1.5 million, could be due to waterborne or foodborne diseases (*84, 88, 89*). In surveys conducted in the United Kingdom, 5–7% of respondents reported having suffered from a foodborne disease during the previous 12 months (*90–92*). In Canada, the estimated figure in the

Table 3. Incidence of foodborne diseases in some industrialized countries, according to surveys or estimates

Year	Country	Percentage of population experiencing a foodborne illness		Reference
1985	Canada	8	(estimate)	*85*
1985	USA	>10	(estimate)	*86, 87, 94, 95*
1991	Netherlands	10	(sentinel study on gastrointestinal diseases)	*84, 88, 89*
1993	Sweden	7	(national survey on suspected foodborne illness)	*83*
1993	New Zealand	9	(national survey on suspected foodborne illness)	*93*
1994	United Kingdom	7	(national survey on suspected foodborne illness)	*90-92*

late 1980s was about 2.2 million cases annually (*85*). In New Zealand, 9% of the surveyed population indicated that they had experienced a suspected foodborne illness in the previous year (*93*).

The dominant problems in industrialized countries are salmonellosis and campylobacteriosis. The incidence of both diseases has increased tremendously during the past decade. Salmonellosis accounts for the greatest proportion of foodborne disease outbreaks and is mostly due to *Salmonella enteritidis,* which is transmitted mainly through contaminated eggs and foods containing eggs and poultry, and *Salmonella typhimurium. S. enteritidis* and *S. typhimurium* account for about 75% of salmonella isolates in the European Salmonella Network, Salm-Net (*97*). From 1985 to 1995, *S. enteritidis* alone caused 582 outbreaks in the USA, making 24 058 people ill, with 2290 cases of hospitalization and 70 deaths (*98*). Poultry, milk and milk products have also been implicated in outbreaks of salmonellosis, as well as of campylobacteriosis. In some countries a great proportion (up to 60% or more) of poultry has been reported to be contaminated with *Salmonella* or *Campylobacter* (*99–102*). For instance, despite a decline in the level of contamination, 33% of the chilled and 41% of the frozen raw chicken produced in the United Kingdom and sold retail in 1993 was found to be contaminated with *Salmonella* (*103*). Some milkborne outbreaks have been caused by recontamination of pasteurized milk. For instance, in 1985 some 170 000–200 000 people were involved in an outbreak of salmonellosis in Illinois, USA, due to contaminated pasteurized milk (*104*). Many outbreaks of salmonellosis and campylobacteriosis are due to the consumption of raw milk and milk products. Although campylobacteriosis does not feature prominently in foodborne disease outbreaks, its incidence is nevertheless very high and in many countries exceeds the incidence of salmonellosis.

Industrialized countries have also been affected by a number of new or newly recognized foodborne diseases such as listeriosis and enterohaemorrhagic *E. coli* infections (see page 14).

An analysis of data from the WHO Surveillance Programme for Control of Foodborne Infections and Intoxications in Europe, covering 21 European countries during 1992–1993, indicated that, where the agent of the foodborne disease outbreak was identified, *Salmonella* caused 84.5% of all outbreaks (*S. enteritidis* 50.9%), *Staphylococcus aureus* 3.5%, *C. perfringens* 3.0%, *C. botulinum* 1.1%, *Trichinella* 1.5%, mushroom intoxication 1.3% and *B. cereus* 1.0% of all outbreaks. All other causative agents accounted for less than 1% (*105, 106*). Table 4 shows the etiology of foodborne disease outbreaks in Latin America and the Caribbean.

Due to rigorous monitoring and to food safety and quality controls by large food manufacturers and retailers, the food supply in industrialized countries is generally safe from chemicals. Nevertheless, accidental contamination or adulteration does occur. In Spain, in 1981–1982, adulterated cooking oil killed more than 800 people and disabled a further 20 000, many permanently

Table 4. Etiology of foodborne disease outbreaks (with known etiology) in Latin America and the Caribbean, 1995–1997

Etiological agent	Percentage of outbreaks	Percentage of cases involved in outbreaks
Bacteria	46.3	83.03
Of which:		
Bacillus cereus	1.3	1.2
Clostridium perfringens	4.2	4.1
Clostridium botulinum	0.4	0.1
Escherichia coli	11.4	7.8
Salmonella	37.0	43.1
Shigella spp.	3.1	21.9
Staphylococcus aureus	36.6	19.5
Vibrio cholerae	4.2	0.9
Vibrio parahaemolyticus	0.2	0.4
Other	1.6	1.0
Total	100.0	100.0
Viruses	1.8	3.7
Parasites	1.8	2.9
Marine toxins	44.2	8.0
Plant toxins	0.4	0.1
Chemical substances	5.4	2.3
Total	**100.0**	**100.0**

Source: Adapted from data provided by the Pan American Institute for Food Protection and Zoonoses, INPPAZ, PAHO/WHO 1998

(*107*). In both Europe and North America, misidentification of mushrooms is one of the leading causes of illness and death from chemical intoxicants.

Trends and under-reporting of foodborne diseases

It is disconcerting that the incidence of foodborne diseases has, in many parts of the world, increased substantially and may continue to increase unless effective measures are taken to prevent it. In Europe, between 1984 and 1990, the incidence increased threefold (*82*). Similar trends have been observed in other parts of the world. For instance, data from New Zealand suggest a 240% increase between 1980 and 1990 (*93*). Figs. 2 and 3 show the situation in the Federal Republic of Germany and in Venezuela. Some governments have taken measures to improve food safety, and as a result, the increase has apparently slowed in some places. Nevertheless, the incidence of foodborne diseases remains very high in most countries.

11

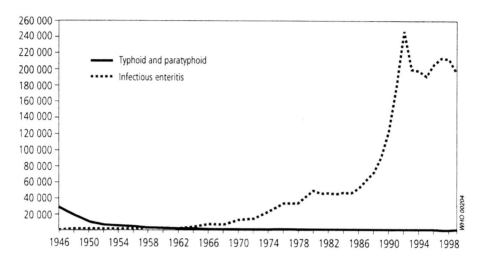

Fig. 2. The incidence of infectious enteritis, typhoid fever and paratyphoid fever in Germany, 1946-1998 (Source of data: Statistiches Bundesamt, Wiesbaden)

Since only a small proportion of cases of foodborne disease actually come to the notice of health services, and even fewer cases are investigated, reported incidence is only the tip of the iceberg; the real number of cases is probably much higher. It is estimated that in industrialized countries less than 10%, or even 1%, of cases are reported (*108*). Some studies in industrialized countries point to an under-reporting factor as high as 350 for certain diseases (*87, 89*). A survey of foodborne disease in Sweden showed that 79 of 1000 persons in the age group 16–74 suffer from one or more episodes of foodborne illness annually, whereas the official figure is 0.25 per 1000 persons (*83*). This indicates an under-reporting factor of 316.

One reason for this high level of under-reporting is that most people suffering from foodborne illness do not seek medical attention. In New Zealand none of the 9% of people surveyed who had suffered from foodborne illness had visited a physician (*93*). In the Swedish survey, 79.5% of people suffering from a foodborne disease did not request medical assistance (*83*). In the Netherlands, only 5% of persons suffering from foodborne illness consulted a physician (*88*). Although similar data are not available from developing countries, there is reason to believe that an even lower proportion of cases, particularly among adults, come to the notice of health services there.

A person's motivation for consulting a physician depends not only on the severity of the illness but also on the perception of the disease and what financial costs are involved. Experience from some countries indicates that if patients

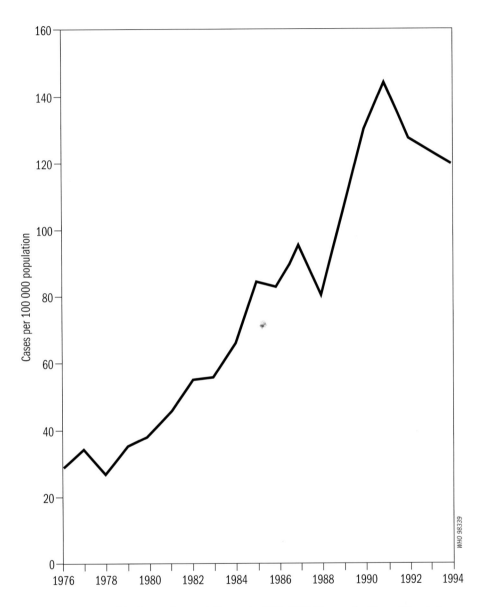

Fig. 3. The incidence of foodborne diseases in Venezuela, 1976–1994 (Source: *Health conditions in the Americas*. Washington, DC, Pan American Health Organization, 1994)

are asked to pay a consultation fee, the number of reported cases of cholera and other diarrhoeal diseases goes down. Lack of recognition of foodborne diseases, misdiagnosis, and lack of laboratory skills or facilities for examining stools are other factors that contribute to under-reporting.

In some industrialized countries, incidence of some foodborne diseases has decreased following specific prevention programmes. For example, the incidence of trichinellosis has decreased significantly in the USA and some other industrialized countries. In the 1940s, an average of 400 cases and 10–15 deaths were reported in the USA each year, but from 1982 to 1986 the number declined to an average of 57 cases per year and a total of three deaths. Freezing of foodstuffs has contributed to the decline in trichinellosis in the USA. Most continuing outbreaks are due to undercooking of pork and game meat.[1] Many occur among immigrants from south-east Asia who eat fermented raw pork. A similar downward trend is also observed in western Europe, with the exception of France where several outbreaks of trichinellosis due to the consumption of horse meat have occurred since 1975 (*109*).

Another disease of which the incidence has decreased tremendously and which has even been eradicated in some countries is brucellosis. This success should be attributed to animal health measures (e.g. immunization of animals) and the pasteurization of milk. Unfortunately, too many cases of brucellosis still occur in developing and some industrialized countries due to consumption or utilization of raw milk or cheese made with raw milk. In France, 54% of some 5000 estimated cases in 1989 (146 cases were reported) were caused by cheese made with raw goat's milk (*110*). In countries of the Mediterranean basin, the Indian subcontinent and parts of Central and South America brucellosis is still highly prevalent (*111*).

Emergence of new or newly recognized types of foodborne diseases

"Emerging" infectious diseases can be defined as infections that have newly appeared in a population, or that have previously existed but due to various factors (such as ecological, environmental, food production, or demographic factors) are rapidly increasing in incidence or geographical range. Some previously unrecognized diseases may also be considered emerging since their recognition is due to increased knowledge or to improved ways of identifying and analysing the disease agent (*112*).

Public health authorities in many countries have been challenged by the emergence of new or newly recognized foodborne pathogens (*112, 113*). Examples are given in Table 5.

---

[1] Larvae present in wild game appear to be relatively resistant to freezing. This may explain many cases of trichinellosis associated with eating game.

Infection with *E. coli* serotype O157:H7 was first described in 1982. Subsequently, it has emerged rapidly as a major cause of bloody diarrhoea and acute renal failure that can be fatal for children and the elderly. Outbreaks of this infection have been reported from Australia, Canada, Japan, the United States and many European countries (*113*). In 1993, a major outbreak of *E. coli* O157:H7 infection affected some 500 people in the north-western states of the USA. Many children developed haemolytic uraemic syndrome and four died as a result (*114*). Another large outbreak caused by this pathogen occurred in Africa, affecting thousands of people; drinking-water and cooked maize were the vehicles for transmission (*115*). In 1996, the largest ever recorded outbreak of *E. coli* O157:H7 occurred in Japan, affecting 6309 schoolchildren and 92 school staff members (*116*). The outbreak resulted in two deaths. The epidemiological investigation identified fresh radish sprouts (*kaiware-daikon*) as the probable cause of the outbreak. Another important outbreak of *E. coli* O157 occurred in Scotland from November 1996 to January 1997. Some 400 people were affected and about 20 elderly people died as a consequence. The outbreak was traced to cold cooked meat (loose or in sandwiches) bought from a local butcher (*117*). Fig. 4 shows the increasing incidence of enterohaemorrhagic *E. coli* infections in the United Kingdom.

Listeria monocytogenes affects particularly vulnerable groups such as immunocompromised individuals, pregnant women, neonates and the elderly (*118*). Outbreaks of listeriosis have been reported from many countries, including Australia, Switzerland and the USA (*119, 120*). Two consecutive outbreaks of *Listeria monocytogenes* in France in 1992 and 1993 were caused by contaminated pork tongue in aspic and rillettes (potted pork); they affected 279 people (with 85 deaths) and 39 people respectively (*120*). Soft cheese and meat paste have been identified as major vehicles of listeriosis. In 1989–1990, meat paste was the source of a major outbreak that affected some 300 victims in the United Kingdom. Soft cheese has been implicated in numerous outbreaks both in Europe and elsewhere. A recent outbreak in France affected 36 persons (*121*). France reported 375 perinatal cases in 1991 and 412 perinatal cases in 1992, accounting for 38% and 31% of total cases respectively (*120*).

Some pathogens have acquired new niches and have posed formerly unrecognized problems. *Salmonella enteritidis*, one of the major causes of foodborne

Table 5. Examples of emerging foodborne pathogens

Enterohaemorrhagic *Escherichia coli*
Listeria monocytogenes
Vibrio cholerae 0139
Salmonella enteritidis
Campylobacter jejuni
Yersinia enterocolitica
Cryptosporidium parvum
Clonorchis sinensis
Opisthorchis viverrini
Cyclospora cayetanensis

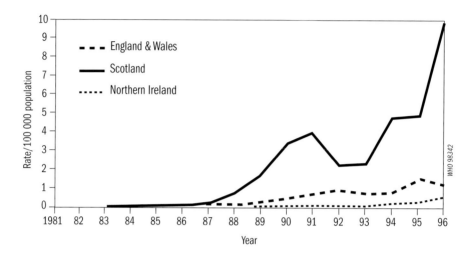

Fig. 4. Increasing incidence of enterohaemorrhagic *E. coli* infection in the United Kingdom (Source: Reproduced by permission of PHLS/CDSC, United Kingdom)

diseases in Europe and the USA, has shown the potential to contaminate yolk of eggs. Intact eggs, which were formerly considered as safe foodstuffs, today require specific vigilance in their preparation.

As the number of immunocompromised persons—particularly AIDS sufferers—has increased, many pathogens of an opportunistic nature (e.g. enterohaemorrhagic *E. coli*, *Cryptosporidium parvum*, *Toxoplasma gondii*) have found new victims in the population.

Cholera has gained new territories. In 1991 it spread to Latin America. A new strain of *V. cholerae* (O139) has also emerged in Bangladesh. A foodborne outbreak of *V. cholerae* O139 Bengal has been reported in British, Canadian and United States tourists visiting Thailand (*122*).

Foodborne trematodes are also emerging as a serious public health problem, partly because of increased awareness of their epidemiology but also because of changes in the food production system which have led to boosting of aquaculture, sometimes under poor sanitary conditions.

International food trade, international travel and migration are also important factors in the emergence or re-emergence (increase in incidence) of certain foodborne diseases (Box 1) (*124*). For example, in some states of the USA the epidemiology of brucellosis has changed from that of an occupational illness to a foodborne illness in the last decade, mainly due to the predilection of Hispanic immigrants for consuming raw milk and cheese made with raw milk. Some diseases may also emerge or re-emerge as a result of changes in diet or food preparation habits. These may change as a result of international travel or international trade in food, and also as a result of nutrition campaigns and recommendations. For instance, public information campaigns in the USA have promoted an increase in the consumption of fruits and vegetables. Consequently, the number of salad bars and food outlets serving fresh fruits and salads have also increased (*125*). Epidemiological data have shown that the proportion of foodborne disease outbreaks related to these products has doubled from 2% during the period 1973–1987 to 5% during 1988–1991 (*126*).

Other emerging problems include diarrhoeal illness due to *Cyclosopora cayetanensis*. In the USA

Box 1. Migration and foodborne diseases(*123*)

In 1991, a 60-year-old man who had emigrated from the Republic of Korea and settled in the USA developed acute hepatitis and renal failure after eating uncooked gall bladder of carp. Although such cases have been recognized in east Asian countries, this was the first reported case in the USA. Such cases raise the question of the education of health workers vis-à-vis exotic foodborne diseases that will increasingly occur with international trade in food and growing migration and travel.

---

between May and mid-July 1996, almost 1000 laboratory-confirmed cases were reported to the Centers for Disease Control and Prevention. The outbreak was attributed to consumption of imported fresh raspberries that had probably been in contact with contaminated water. The route of transmission of cyclospora needs to be elucidated, but it is believed that the parasites may be transmitted through the faecal–oral route (*127*). Some emerging diseases have characteristics that suggest they might be foodborne although adequate data are not available to confirm this. An example is *Helicobacter pylori* infection. The faecal–oral route has been considered one of the possible routes of transmission and therefore foodborne transmission through contamination with faecal matter has been also considered a possibility. In Santiago, Chile, consumption of raw vegetables fertilized with human faeces was found to be a risk factor for this infection (*128*). *Helicobacter pylori* causes peptic ulcer disease and can lead to severe anaemia due to chronic gastric blood loss. Infection may also cause gastric carcinoma (*113, 129*).

Health consequences of foodborne diseases

Except for a few diseases such as botulism, brucellosis and listeriosis, foodborne diseases are often viewed as mild and self-limiting. While this may sometimes be true, in many cases the health consequences can be serious, even life-threatening. False perception has in part contributed to the lack of attention paid to this problem.

The health consequences of foodborne diseases vary according to the pathogen, stage of treatment and duration, as well as age and other factors that define a person's resistance and susceptibility. Acute symptoms include diarrhoea, nausea, vomiting, abdominal pain, cramps, fever and jaundice. In most cases immunocompetent persons recover within a few days or a few weeks. In some cases, however, particularly among vulnerable groups (e.g. the elderly, infants, young children, pregnant women, and malnourished, immunocompromised persons), some foodborne diseases may be fatal, especially when adequate treatment is not available.

Some foodborne infections can lead to serious complications that affect the cardiovascular, renal, articular, respiratory or immune systems (Table 6) (*130*). Among vulnerable groups, these health effects may be even more serious. In a survey of 32 448 cases of foodborne disease in the Russian Federation, chronic health effects occurred in over 11% of patients, with hypertension and cholelithiasis being the most frequent. A number of patients also developed myocardial infarction (*131*).

Examples of severe complications associated with foodborne illness are reactive arthritis and rheumatoid syndromes, meningitis, endocarditis, Reiter syndrome, Guillain–Barré syndrome and haemolytic uraemic syndrome (*132, 133*). For instance, salmonellosis has been reported to cause reactive arthritis in some subjects. In the milkborne salmonellosis outbreak that occurred in Illinois in 1985, some 2% of patients developed reactive arthritis as a result (*104*).

A proportion of patients, particularly children, who are affected by *E. coli* O157:H7 may develop haemolytic uraemic syndrome which is characterized by acute renal failure. The manifestations of listeriosis may include septicaemia, meningitis, encephalitis, osteomyelitis and endocarditis; in pregnant women, the disease may lead to abortion, stillbirth or malformation of the fetus. The overall fatality rate is about 30%. In an outbreak of listeriosis in pregnant women in Western Australia, the fatality rate of infected fetuses was as high as 50% (*134*).

Transplacental infections of *Toxoplasma gondii* may occur in some 45% of infected pregnant women (*135*). In 10–20% of nonfatal morbidity, infants may suffer from damage to the central nervous system and retinochoroiditis leading to blindness (*136*). It is believed that infected but asymptomatic infants may also develop sequelae, most commonly retinochoroiditis, later in life (*137, 138*). It is estimated that globally in about three out of every 1000 pregnancies the fetus/infant is affected by toxoplasmosis (*139*).

Infections due to *Vibrio vulnificus* may be present as fulminant septicaemia, often complicated with necrotizing cutaneous lesions. According to some studies, the case fatality rate for patients with pre-existing liver disease is 63% and is 23% for those without liver disease (*140*).

Cysticercosis, infection with the larval stage of *Taenia solium*, is common particularly in South and Central America and may lead to cerebral lesions. The liver flukes *Opisthorchis viverrini* and *Clonorchis sinensis* cause mechanical

Table 6. Complications of and chronic health effects associated with foodborne infections (Source: Adapted with permission from *130*)

Bacterial and parasitic infection transmitted by foods	Complication/sequelae
Bacterial infections	
Aeromonas hydrophila enteritis[a]	Bronchopneumonia, cholecystitis
Brucellosis	Aortitis, epididymo-orchitis, meningitis, pericarditis, spondylitis
Campylobacteriosis	Arthritis, carditis, cholecystitis, colitis, endocarditis, erythema nodosum, Guillain-Barré syndrome, haemolyticuraemic syndrome, meningitis, pancreatitis, septicaemia
Escherichia coli (EHEC[b]-types) enteritis	Erythema nodosum, haemolyticuraemic syndrome, seronegative arthropathy, thrombotic thrombocytopenic purpura
Listeriosis	Meningitis
Q-fever	Endocarditis, granulomatous hepatitis
Salmonellosis	Aortitis, cholecystitis, colitis, endocarditis, epididymo-orchitis, meningitis, myocarditis, osteomyelitis, pancreatitis, Reiter disease, rheumatoid syndromes, septicaemia, splenic abscesses, thyroiditis, septic arthritis (sickle-cell anaemic persons)
Shigellosis	Erythema nodosum, haemolyticuraemic syndrome, peripheral neuropathy, pneumonia, Reiter disease, septicaemia, splenic abscesses, synovitis
Vibrio parahaemolyticus enteritis	Septicaemia
Yersiniosis	Arthritis, cholangitis, erythema nodosum, hepatic and splenic abscesses, lymphadenitis, pneumonia, pyomyositis, Reiter disease, septicaemia, spondylitis, Still disease
Parasitic infection	
Cryptosporidiosis[c]	Severe diarrhoea, prolonged and sometimes fatal
Giardiasis[c]	Cholangitis, dystrophy, joint symptoms, lymphoidal hyperplasia
Taeniasis	Arthritis, cysticercosis (*T. solium*)
Toxoplasmosis	Encephalitis and other central nervous system diseases, pancarditis, polymyositis
Trematodiasis	Liver cancer
Trichinosis	Cardiac dysfunction, neurological sequelae

[a] Suspected to be foodborne or waterborne.
[b] Enterohaemorrhagic *E. coli*.
[c] Waterborne.

obstruction of the biliary tract and recurrent pyogenic cholangitis; they are carcinogenic to humans (*55*).

Repeated episodes of foodborne disease can lead to malnutrition, with serious impact on the growth and immune system of infants and children. The infant whose resistance is compromised becomes more vulnerable to other diseases (including respiratory infections) and is subsequently caught in a vicious cycle of malnutrition and infection (Fig. 5). Many infants and children do not survive in these circumstances. Annually, 12–13 million children under the age of five years die due to the associated effects of malnutrition and infections (*3*).

Serious health consequences have been reported when foods with chemical contaminants such as heavy metals (i.e. methyl mercury, lead and cadmium) have been ingested over extended periods. Lead affects haematopoiesis, renal function and the nervous system. Mercury has also serious effects on the nervous system. Both mercury and lead are particularly dangerous for pregnant women.

Cost of foodborne diseases

In addition to death and ill-health caused by foodborne diseases, tremendous economic costs are incurred by individuals, families, health care systems and society, as well as by commercial enterprises. These include loss of income due to absenteeism, the cost of medical care, the cost of investigating foodborne disease outbreaks, loss of income due to closure of businesses, legal costs and fines (Box 2) (*141–143*).

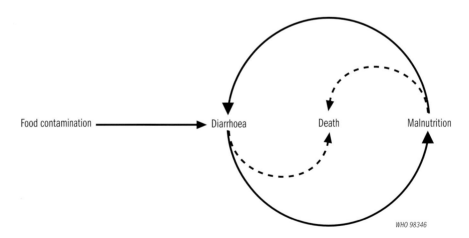

WHO 98346

Fig. 5. Diarrhoea and malnutrition combine to form a cycle leading to declining health status and death (Source: 5)

The national cost of salmonellosis in England and Wales in 1992 has been estimated at between £350 million and £502 million with an average cost per case of between £789 and £861. Over 73% of costs were direct costs associated with treatment and investigation of cases and costs to the economy from sickness-related absence from work. The social cost of loss of production was the largest component of the total (*143*).

Foodborne illnesses are a leading reason for absenteeism. According to a local magazine, a 1992 survey in Hong Kong showed that up to 30% of workers take days off during the year because of foodborne illness (*144*). A survey in Sweden found that some 160 000 persons stayed home from work for a total of around 300 000 days in one year (*83*).

In the USA, the total annual cost of salmonellosis has been calculated at about US$ 4 million, with an average cost per case of US$ 1350. In addition, the costs of foodborne hepatitis A and Norwalk agent infection have been estimated at US$ 5000 and US$ 887 respectively (*62, 130*).

In Argentina, treatment of a case of diarrhoea in a government hospital, with five days' hospitalization, has been estimated to cost about US$ 2000.

For a food service establishment, the effects of an outbreak of foodborne illness may be devastating. An analysis of economic losses associated with food service establishments in Canada and the USA showed that costs ranged from US$ 16 690 to over US$ 1 million per outbreak with an average of US$ 788 per individual affected (*145*). These estimations were made in 1985; the figure today will be certainly much higher. Table 7 shows the cost of foodborne diseases in a number of countries (*146–162*).

Cost estimates for foodborne diseases are not available from developing countries. However, episodes of diarrhoeal disease, which in some countries affect children on average 10 times during the first year of life, are undoubtedly one of the most frequent reasons for the hospitalization of children. In

---

Box 2. Economic losses associated with foodborne diseases (Adapted from *141*)

■ **Costs of investigations and testing**

■ **Health care costs**
- general practitioner costs
- hospital costs
- costs of medicines
- ambulance costs.

■ **Costs to families and societies**
- costs attributable to loss of productivity and absenteeism
- costs attributable to pain, suffering and death
- direct costs of illness to families.

■ **Costs to commercial enterprises**
- closure of business
- fines and legal pursuit
- loss of customers due to lost reputation
- condemnation of food implicated in outbreaks.

Table 7. Annual incidence and cost of foodborne illnesses in selected countries according to different estimates

Disease	Country	Incidence (cases/year)	Cost (in million US$)	Reference
Foodborne illness	Canada (1985)	2.2 million	1335	*146*
Bacterial foodborne illness	Canada	1 million	1100	*147*
Foodborne illness	Croatia (1986–92)	8500 (average reported cases per year)	1.3	*148*
Foodborne illness	New Zealand (1991)		>50	*149*
Foodborne illness	USA	12.6 million	8400	*150*
Foodborne illness	USA	33 million	7700	*151*
Foodborne diarrhoeal diseases	USA	24–81 million		*152*
Bacterial foodborne illness	USA (1987)	6.3 million	4800	*153*
Intestinal infectious diseases	USA (1985)	99 million (1980)	23 000	*154*
Salmonellosis	Croatia (1986–92)	3860 (average reported cases per year)	1.1	*155*
Salmonellosis	England and Wales (1991)	23 000	64–80	*156*
Salmonellosis	USA (1987)	1 920 000	1344	*153*
Salmonellosis	USA (1978–82)	2 960 000	3991	*150*
Campylobacteriosis	USA (1987)	2 100 000	1470	*153*
Campylobacteriosis	USA (1978–82)	170 000	156	*150*
S. aureus intoxication	USA (1978–82)	1 155 000	1500	*150*
E. coli O157:H7 infection	USA (1978–82)	25 000	84	*150*
E. coli O157:H7 infection	USA (1992)	7700–20 500	217–579	*157*
Listeriosis	USA (1987)	1580	213	*153*
Listeriosis	USA (1986)	1860	480	*158*
Listeriosis	USA (1978–82)	25 000	313	*150*
Trichinellosis	USA (1978–82)	40 000	144	*150*
Toxoplasmosis	USA (1978–82)	1 435 400	445	*150*
Congenital toxoplasmosis	USA (1992)		2628	*159*
Cysticercosis	Mexico (1992)	52 620	195	*160*
Opisthorchiasis	Thailand (1992)		99.9	*161*
Hepatitis A	USA	143 000	200	*165*
Hepatitis A	Worldwide	>1.4 million	1500–3000	*165*

some areas, diarrhoeal disease accounts for 30% or more of paediatric hospitalization (*163*). In Bangladesh, diarrhoeal syndromes have been reported to account for 52% of paediatric hospitalizations (*164, 165*). A study of costs associated with the treatment of inpatients aged under 5 years in Cuba and the Philippines indicated an average cost per case of treatment in the medical centre of around US$ 50 in 1989. The total estimated cost of treatment in households amounted to over 6 million pesos (US$ 276 128) (*166*). Although the cost of treatment of a similar case in the industrialized countries would have been up to 10 times greater, one must bear in mind the frail economy of these countries, the higher rate of incidence, and the fact that these data represent only the cost of treatment of a segment of the population. Overall, these costs represent a tremendous economic burden in developing countries.

At national level, epidemics of foodborne diseases may affect tourism and the food trade. During 1991, the outbreak of cholera cost Peru more than US$ 700 million in loss of exports of fish and fishery products. In the three months following the start of the epidemic US$ 70 million were lost due to the closure of food service establishments and the decrease in tourism (*167*).

Factors leading to the prevalence of foodborne diseases

Industrialization, urbanization and changing lifestyle

As a result of industrialization and urbanization, the food chain has become longer and more complex. Opportunities for the contamination of food have increased. Improved standards of living, particularly in middle-income and high-income groups, have led to an increase in the consumption of food of animal origin. This in turn has led to a rise in the risk of exposure to pathogens transmitted in milk, meat and poultry. The extensive demand for food of animal origin has in turn boosted the mass breeding and raising of animals with the resulting risk that many of these animals may be subclinically infected with foodborne pathogens such as *Salmonella* and *Campylobacter*.

A consequence of industrialization and mass production of food is that whenever outbreaks occur as a result of failures during food processing in food industries, a large number of people may be at risk. Where the system of foodborne disease surveillance and investigation is poor, outbreaks can affect even more people since identification of the source and containment of the outbreak take longer.

With urbanization and industrialization, lifestyles are changing. Mothers who have taken up jobs outside the home do not always bear complete responsibility for the preparation of family meals. Other family members, sometimes less experienced, or ill-trained domestic helpers are involved in preparing meals. Consequently, traditional methods of food preparation that in the past ensured the safety of food have tended to disappear in recent years. A survey in the United Kingdom showed that 81% of those aged 55 years or over always ensure that food is served hot and eaten immediately after serving, compared to 54% of those aged under 24 years.

Changes in lifestyle also mean that in some societies there are now many persons living alone and eating "convenience" pre-prepared foods (either catered or leftovers). Many people also eat more frequently in food service establishments (restaurants, canteens, etc.), or buy their food from street food vendors. In middle-income and high-income countries, the number of food service and catering establishments has increased tremendously. In France, for instance, over 6000 million meals are served annually in these places (*109*). In the USA from 1972 to 1989, the number of restaurants increased from 112 000 to 161 000 and the number of fast-food restaurants doubled from 73 000 to more than 146 000 (*168*). Persons involved in the preparation of food in such establishments may lack formal education or training in food safety and many may not even know the basics of food hygiene. As women have entered the workforce, the number of children attending child care facilities has increased in many places during the past decade. For example, 11 million children attend these facilities in the USA (*169*). In industrialized countries, a growing number of elderly persons are also living in care institutions.

Socioeconomic factors, increased unemployment, urbanization and tourism have also led to rapid expansion in street food vending in recent years. Food prepared and sold by street food vendors is sometimes of poor hygienic standard and may occasionally be adulterated. In a survey of food sold by 34 street food vendors in Sousse, Tunisia, it was found that only 26% of food samples were of satisfactory quality (*170*). Outbreaks of severe foodborne intoxications involving some hundreds of schoolchildren have repeatedly been reported in some African countries (*171*). Street food has also been recognized as an important vehicle for the transmission of cholera and other foodborne diseases in Asia and Latin America (*33, 38, 172–175*).

Changing population

The proportion of the population susceptible to foodborne infections is increasing. In particular, the population is growing older as life expectancy increases. This is all the more important in countries where the population benefits from better nutrition, medical care and welfare. The number of persons immunocompromised by HIV infection, malignancy and immunosuppressive treatment has also increased. War, famine and natural disasters such as earthquakes and floods lead to increased malnutrition and precipitate conditions in which foodborne diseases thrive (*130*). Table 8 shows the factors that increase the risk or severity of foodborne illness.

Table 8. Factors increasing the risk of foodborne infection or the severity of illness (Source: Reproduced with permission from *130*)

Factors	Reasons
Microbial factors	
Type and strain of pathogen ingested	Some pathogens and strains more virulent than others
Quantity of pathogens ingested	Higher numbers ingested may increase severity of illness and/or shorten onset time
Host factors	
Age less than 5 years	Lack of developed immune systems, smaller infective dose-by-weight required
Age greater than 50 or 60 years (depending on pathogen)	Immune systems failing, weakened by chronic ailments, occurring as early as 50 to 60 years of age
Pregnancy	Altered immunity during pregnancy
Hospitalized persons	Immune systems weakened by other diseases or injuries, or at risk of exposure to antibiotic-resistant strains
Concomitant infections	Overloaded or damaged immune systems
Consumption of antibiotics	Alteration of normal intestinal microflora
Excessive iron in blood	Iron in blood serving as nutrient for certain organisms
Reduced liver/kidney function (alcoholism)	Reduced digestion capabilities, altered blood-iron concentrations
Possession of certain human antigenic determinants duplicated or easily mimicked by microorganisms	Predisposition to chronic illnesses (sequelae)
Surgical removal of portions of stomach or intestines	Reduction in normal defensive systems against infection
Immunocompromised individuals including those on chemotherapy or radiation therapy; recipients of organ transplants taking immunocompromising drugs; persons with leukaemia, AIDS, or other illnesses	Immune system inadequate to prevent infection
Stress	Body metabolism changes allowing easier establishment of pathogens, or lower dose of toxin required for illness
Poor hygiene	Increased likelihood of ingestion of pathogens

Table 8. *Continued*

Factors	Reasons
Diet-related factors	
Nutritional deficiencies either through poor absorption of food (mostly ill or elderly persons) or unavailability of adequate food supply (undernourished persons)	Inadequate strength to build up resistance and/or consumption of poor-quality food ingredients, which may contain pathogens
Consumption of antacids	Increased pH of stomach
Consumption of large volume of liquids including water	Dilution of acids in the stomach and rapid transit through the stomach
Ingestion of fatty foods (such as chocolate, cheese, hamburger) containing pathogens	Protection of pathogens by the fat against stomach acids
Other factors	
Geographical location	Likelihood of exposure to endemic virulent strains, limited food and water supply, varied distribution of organisms in water and soil

International trade in food and feed

International trade in food and animal feed has contributed to the spread of diseases to new areas. For instance, some strains of *Salmonella* have been introduced into North America and Europe through contaminated feeds of animal and vegetable origin imported from tropical and subtropical regions. Animals given these feeds have, in turn, contaminated the environment (soil, rivers, surface water and, subsequently, insects, rodents and birds) with their faeces. The microorganisms have established themselves widely in the environment and in domestic and wild animals. A large outbreak of *Salmonella typhi* infection occurred in Aberdeen, United Kingdom, following the importation of canned corned beef from Argentina (*176*). In 1995, outbreaks of shigellosis occurred in several northern European countries as a result of the importation of iceberg lettuce contaminated with *Shigella sonnei* from Spain (*177*). Due to lack of epidemiological surveillance of foodborne diseases it is difficult to trace outbreaks of foodborne disease in developing countries to imported food. However, it can be assumed that such outbreaks occur frequently.

Polluted environment, poverty and lack of food preparation facilities

A polluted environment, poverty and lack of facilities for the preparation of safe food are interrelated factors which compromise food safety in poor social settings. Lack of water, sanitation, facilities for cold storage and fuel for cooking (gas, wood, electricity) hamper safe food preparation and lead to conditions that favour foodborne diseases. Constraints such as lack of fuel or time for cooking may lead households to adopt food preparation and storage practices that may be detrimental to child health. It is often observed that, in order to save fuel or time, food is prepared in larger quantities than needed for one meal and then stored for subsequent meal times, often at ambient temperature. Sometimes such food may remain insufficiently cooked. Because of the shortage of fuel, the stored food may be served cold or be inadequately reheated, contributing to the increased risk of foodborne diarrhoeal disease. During the hot season—which coincides with an increase in the rate of many diarrhoeal diseases—storage of food at ambient temperature creates an even greater risk as higher temperature is even more favourable to the growth of microorganisms (*3*).

Tourism

Hundreds of millions of travellers cross international borders every year, and the number is increasing. The World Tourism Organization estimated tourist arrivals worldwide in 1996 at 592 million (excluding one-day trips). This figure is expected to double over the next 10 years and by 2010 over 1000 million people a year will be making international trips (*178*).

International travel now has implications in terms of foodborne disease. One relates to the health of the travellers themselves who run a greater risk of being exposed to foodborne disease agents. For instance, it has been demonstrated that European tourists who visit Mediterranean countries run a risk of developing diarrhoea that is 20 times the risk they would run in their own country (*179*). It is estimated that, depending on the area visited, 20–50% of travellers run the risk of contracting diarrhoea (*107, 180*). At some destinations a traveller's risk of contracting diarrhoea has been reported to be over 60% (Fig. 6) (*181*).

The increased risk of foodborne disease in travellers results from the fact that travellers are often obliged to eat in restaurants and hotels, buy their meals from street vendors—who may not always observe the rules of food hygiene—or prepare their food on campsites where conditions of hygiene are rudimentary. However, in many instances travellers do not take the necessary precautions. In a study of some 662 travellers to Kenya, Maldives and Sri Lanka, it was found that the incidence of diarrhoea (19.5%) was in proportion to the number of dietary mistakes made and the most

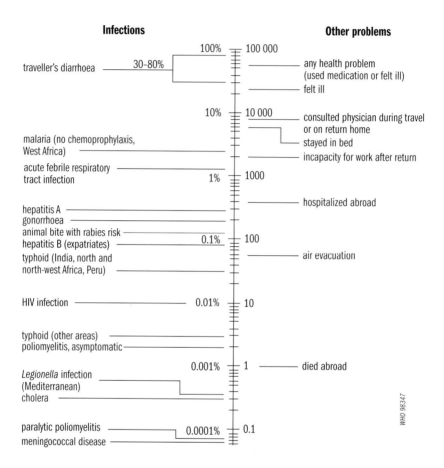

Fig. 6. Estimated monthly incidence of health problems per 100 000 travellers to tropical areas (*180*)

dangerous foods were those that travellers were traditionally recommended to avoid (*182*).

Another implication of international travel, as well as of migration, is the spread of foodborne diseases to other countries. Travellers may become infected abroad and "import" a disease to their country of residence, or they may be subclinically infected and become the source of secondary infections on their return home. In some countries the relative importance of imported cases of foodborne disease may be considerable (Fig. 7). For instance, it is estimated that 80–90% of cases of salmonellosis in Scandinavian countries are imported (*183*). A fivefold increase of shigellosis in the USA between the 1970s and the 1980s has been linked to travel to Mexico (*184*). Up to 80% of typhoid fever in some countries is estimated to be travel-related, and the proportion of travel-related typhoid fever has increased considerably in the past years (*185, 186*)

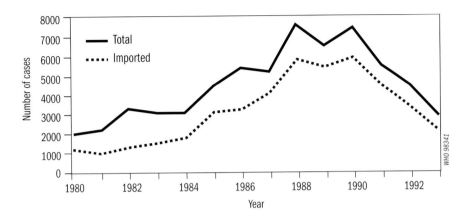

Fig. 7. Human salmonella isolations, Finland. Decrease in the number of salmonellosis cases was due to decrease in number of travellers (Source: Reproduced with permission from *183*)

Knowledge, beliefs and practices of food handlers and consumers

The most important factors in the prevalence of foodborne illnesses are the lack of knowledge on the part of food handlers or consumers and negligence (despite knowledge) in safe food-handling. Surveys of foodborne disease outbreaks worldwide have shown that most cases of foodborne disease occur as the result of an error in handling food during preparation, whether in homes, in food service and catering establishments, in the canteens of hospitals, schools or the military (Box 3), or at banquets and parties. Most cases of foodborne disease could have been avoided—even when the original foodstuff was contaminated—if the food handlers had been better trained in food safety (*106, 187–189*).

A five-year study of foodborne diseases in Saudi Arabia indicated an incidence rate of 22 cases per 100 000 persons. In 56.7% of incidents food was incorrectly handled in the home. Workers' camps and food service establishments were also major sites of foodborne disease outbreaks (*190*). Table 9 shows the sites of foodborne disease outbreaks in Poland, indicating that most outbreaks occur as a result of mishandling during food preparation. A similar situation is reported from other countries, including industrialized countries (*106*). In developing countries, street food vendors are another important source of foodborne diseases (*34, 39, 170–175*).

Food served on aircraft and cruise ships has also been implicated in outbreaks of foodborne disease (*193–207*). Table 10 shows some examples of documented outbreaks of foodborne diseases traced to aircraft. Table 11 provides selected examples of outbreaks where schoolchildren have been affected. It points to the need for more hygienic handling of food served to children (*208–225*). The outbreaks presented in Table 11 are only a small fraction of

29

the outbreaks that have affected children.

Worldwide, surveys of foodborne disease outbreaks indicate that most outbreaks result from food-handling leading to contamination with and/or survival and growth of microorganisms. For example, the following errors in food-handling have been recognized as the major sources of foodborne disease outbreaks in Israel (*106*):

- *Contamination with microorganism:*
  — use of contaminated equipment;
  — contamination by infected person;
  — use of contaminated raw ingredient;
  — cross-contamination;
  — addition of toxic chemicals or use of foods containing natural toxicants.

Box 3. Diarrhoeal diseases in the military

Diarrhoeal diseases have had a profound impact on military operations throughout history. In American history up to the 1940s, more military deaths were due to diarrhoea than to injuries inflicted in war. By the Second World War, mortality due to diarrhoeal diseases decreased. However, they remained a major cause of morbidity (*191*).

Diarrhoeal diseases due to food contamination still occur in armies. During a five-year period from 1985 to 1989, some 162 outbreaks of foodborne diseases occurred in the army in France, affecting some 8970 persons (*192*).

Table 9. Outbreaks of foodborne diseases in Poland 1990–1992 according to site of occurrence (Source of data: *106*)

Place	Year				
	1990 No.	1991 No.	1992 No.	1990–92	
				No.	% of outbreaks
Restaurant, bar, café	61	53	60	174	8.2
Canteen	13	12	13	38	1.8
School, kindergarten	42	29	38	109	5.1
Medical care facilities (hospital, nursery)	31	23	24	78	3.7
Private home	538	546	437	1521	71.4
Vacation centre	16	14	12	42	2.0
Other	33	33	16	82	3.8
Various places (2 or more)	13	29	40	82	3.8
Not known	5	–	–	5	0.2
Total	**752**	**739**	**640**	**2131**	**100.0**

Table 10. Examples of documented foodborne disease outbreaks traced to airlines

Year	Agent	Implicated food	Total no. of cases (confirmed/ probable)	Origin	Reference
1970	*Clostridium perfringens*	Turkey	25	Atlanta, USA	*193*
1971	*Shigella*	Seafood cocktail	19	Bermuda	*194*
1972	*Vibrio parahaemolyticus*	Seafood appetizer	12	Bangkok, Thailand	*195*
1972	*Vibrio cholerae*	Appetizer	47	Bahrain	*13*
1973	*Vibrio cholerae*	Cold asparagus & egg salad	66	Bahrain	*196*
1973	*Salmonella*	Breakfast	>17	Denver, USA	*197*
1975	*Staphylococcus aureus*	Ham	197	Anchorage, USA	*198*
1976	*Salmonella brandenburg*	Multiple items	290	Paris, France	*199*
1976	*Staphylococcus aureus*	Cream cakes	28	Rio de Janeiro, Brazil	*200*
1982	*Staphylococcus aureus*	Custard	16	Lisbon, Portugal	*197*
1983	*Salmonella enteriditis*	Swiss steak	12	New York, USA	*197*
1983	*Shigella*		42	Acapulco, Mexico	*197*
1984	*Salmonella*	Glaze on savoury pastries	1000	London, United Kingdom	*201*
1986	*Salmonella infantis*	Multiple items	91	Vantaa, Finland	*202*
1988	*Shigella*	Cold food items	240	Minnesota, USA	*203*
1989	*Salmonella enteriditis*	Multiple items	71	Spain/Finland	*204*
1991	*Staphylococcus aureus*	Chocolate cake	26	Illinois, USA	*205*
1991	Norwalk-like agent	Commercial orange juice	3050	Melbourne, Australia	*206*
1992	*Vibrio cholerae*	Cold seafood salad	75	Buenos Aires, Argentina	*207*

- *Survival of microorganism:*
  — inadequate heating;
  — inadequate cooking.

- *Growth of microorganism:*
  — inadequate refrigeration;
  — inadequate cooling;
  — keeping food insufficiently hot.

Table 11. Selected examples of documented cases of foodborne diseases affecting schoolchildren or college students

Year	Country	Agent	Implicated or suspected food	Cases children (adults)	Reference
1980	Côte d'Ivoire	Unknown	Unknown (presumably street food)	150	208
1983	Malaysia	*Staphylococcus aureus*	Fried noodles	48	209
1988	USA	*E. coli* O157:H7	Meat pies	32[a]	210
1989	India	*E. coli*	Unknown	76	211
1989	Gambia	*Salmonella typhi*	Unknown	26[b](2)	212
1990	Côte d'Ivoire	Unknown	Unknown (presumably street food)	200	208
1990	USA	*Staphylococcus aureus*	Ham	100	213
1991	USA	*Salmonella javiana*	Watermelon	26[a]	214
1991	Japan	*Astrovirus*	Unknown	>4700[c]	215
1992	Saudi Arabia	*Salmonella typhi*	Cake with cream topping	18(1)	216
1992	Russian Federation	*Staphylococcus aureus*	Unknown	30(2)	217
1993	Russian Federation	*Staphylococcus aureus*	Mixed food items	57(3)	218
1993	USA	*Bacillus cereus*	Chicken fried rice	12(2)	219
1994	Japan	*Yersinia pseudotuberculosis*	Unknown	725(7)	220
1995	UK	*Campylobacter jejuni*	Milk	8[c]	221
1995	UK	*Cryptosporidium*	Milk	48	222
1995	USA	*Clostridium perfringens*	Gravy on turkey	22(18)	223
1996	Japan	*E. coli* O157:H7	Radish sprouts	6309[a](92)	224
1997	Indonesia	Unknown	Green-bean porridge	152	225

[a] Secondary cases excluded.
[b] Seven of these children, also affected by the outbreak, were outside the school feeding programme.
[c] A number of adults are included.

Many instances of foodborne disease occur as a result of consumption of hazardous foods, such as raw seafood, raw or undercooked animal products, or foods contaminated with naturally occurring toxins (toxic mushrooms, mouldy foods). Sometimes culture or tradition may encourage such practices. In many countries, there is a predilection to consume raw seafood (e.g. sushi and sashimi in Japan, raw oysters worldwide). Yet these foods are important vehicles for pathogens such as *Vibrio parahaemolyticus* and *Vibrio vulnificus*, small round viruses and hepatitis A virus. *V. parahaemolyticus* is second to salmonellosis as the leading cause of foodborne illness in Japan with thousands of cases reported each year. Some 5849 cases were reported in Japan in 1994. Fish, shellfish and their products account for about one-third of cases (*226*). *V. vulnificus* from raw oysters has been recognized as the leading cause of reported deaths from foodborne illness in Florida, USA (*140*).

Cultural beliefs and rituals may also have major implications for the preparation of food. For instance, in some cultures babies' stools are not considered dirty and therefore mothers may not wash their hands after cleaning the baby and before preparing food. Similarly, in some Latin American countries, exposing hot hands to cold water is believed to cause cramps and rheumatism, so people refrain from washing them, often for many hours (*227*).

Prevention of foodborne diseases

Prevention of foodborne illnesses requires a multisectoral effort by governments, food industries and consumers. The prevention strategy comprises regulatory measures, educational activities, and the surveillance of foodborne diseases and monitoring of contaminants (*167, 228*).

Regulatory measures

Governments have to ensure that up-to-date food legislation, relevant to prevailing national problems, is in place and is properly enforced. This can be achieved by mandatory compliance or voluntary programmes (*229*). A policy of mandatory compliance is the enforcement of the law, checking compliance with it by inspection and laboratory analysis, and imposing penalties if it is violated. Voluntary programmes, on the other hand, promote good agricultural and manufacturing practices and the application of a modern method of food safety assurance, i.e. The Hazard Analysis Critical Control Point system (HACCP). In this regard, industry and trade, including primary industry (agriculture and fishing) have the responsibility to follow accepted codes of hygienic practice and to comply with laws and regulations. The food industry should recognize the importance of food safety and should seek the means to ensure the safety of its products, such as by the application of the HACCP system which is now internationally recognized as the reference for food safety assurance (*230*).

Educational measures

A complementary but integral approach to prevention of foodborne illnesses is the education and training of food handlers and consumers in food safety. The importance of this subject is discussed at length in the next chapter.

Surveillance

All efforts for ensuring food safety depend on the systematic collection of information on current food-related health problems and recent advances in science and technology. The information obtained through such activities will help in learning about the epidemiology of foodborne diseases, formulating appropriate policies, and prioritizing and evaluating interventions (*124*).

References

1. *Health consequences of biological contamination and chemicals in food. Report of the Panel on Food and Agriculture, WHO Commission on Health and Environment.* Geneva, World Health Organization, 1992 (unpublished document WHO/EHE/92.2; available on request from Department of Protection of the Human Environment, World Health Organization, 1211 Geneva 27, Switzerland).

2. *Ninth programme report 1992–1993: Programme for control of diarrhoeal diseases.* Geneva, World Health Organization, 1994 (unpublished document WHO/CDD/94.46; available on request from Department of Child and Adolescent Health and Development, World Health Organization, 1211 Geneva 27, Switzerland).

3. Motarjemi Y et al. Contaminated weaning food: a major risk factor for diarrhoea and associated malnutrition. *Bulletin of the World Health Organization*, 1993, 71(1):79–92.

4. Esrey SA, Feachem RG. *Interventions for the control of diarrhoeal diseases among young children. Promotion of food hygiene.* Geneva, World Health Organization, 1989 (unpublished document WHO/CDD/89.30; available on request from Department of Child and Adolescent Health and Development, World Health Organization, 1211 Geneva 27, Switzerland).

5. *Readings on diarrhoea. A student manual.* Geneva, World Health Organization, 1992.

6. Wagner EG, Lacroix JN. *Excreta disposal for rural areas and small communities.* Geneva, World Health Organization, 1958 (WHO Monograph Series, No. 39).

7. Cholera in 1993. *Weekly epidemiological record*, 1994, 69(28):205–212.

8. Quevedo F. Foods and cholera. In: Pestana de Castro AF, Almeida WF, eds. *Cholera on the American continents.* Washington, DC, International Life Science Institute (ILSI) Press, 1993.

9. Albert J, Neira M, Motarjemi Y. The role of food in the epidemiology of cholera. *World health statistics quarterly*, 1997, 50(1/2):111–118.

10. Felsenfeld O. *Survival of cholera vibrios on food: practical implications and methods of study.* Geneva, World Health Organization, 1972 (unpublished document BD/cholera/72.1; available on request from Department of Communicable Disease Surveillance and Response, World Health Organization, 1211 Geneva 27, Switzerland).

11. Teng PH. The role of foods in the transmission of cholera. In: Bushnell QA, Brookhyser CS, eds. *Proceeding of Cholera Research Symposium, Honolulu, Hawaii.*

Washington, DC, US Department of Health, Education and Welfare, 1965:328–331.

12. Fattal B, Yekutiel P, Shuval HI. Cholera outbreak in Jerusalem 1970 revisited; the evidence for transmission by wastewater irrigated vegetables. In: Goldsmith JR, ed. *Environmental epidemiology: epidemiological investigation of community environmental health problems.* Boca Raton, FL, CRC Press, 1986.

13. Sutton RGA. An outbreak of cholera in Australia due to food served in flight on an international aircraft. *Journal of hygiene*, 1974, 72:441–451.

14. Baine WB et al. Epidemiology of cholera in Italy in 1973. *Lancet*, 1974, 2(7893):1370–1374.

15. Blake PA et al. Cholera in Portugal, 1974: II—Transmission by bottled mineral water. *American journal of epidemiology*, 1977, 105(4):344–348.

16. Blake PA et al. Cholera in Portugal, 1974: I—Modes of transmission. *American journal of epidemiology*, 1977, 105(4):337–343.

17. Haddock R. Cholera in a Pacific Island. *Journal of diarrhoeal disease research*, 1987, 5(3):181–183.

18. McIntyre RC et al. Modes of transmission of cholera in a newly infected population on an atoll: implications for control measures. *Lancet*, 1979, 1(8111):311–314.

19. Khan MU et al. Vibriocidal titre in cholera cases and contacts: its value in assessing endemicity of or susceptibility to cholera. *Tropical and geographical medicine*, 1987, 30:271–275.

20. Blake PA et al. Cholera—a possible endemic focus in the United States. *New England journal of medicine*, 1980, 302(6):305–309.

21. Gunn RA et al. Bottle feeding as a risk factor for cholera in infants. *Lancet*, 1979, 2(8145):730–732.

22. Fukumi H. Epidemiological aspects on the cholera outbreak in Japan originating from wedding dinner parties in Ikenohata Bunka Center, Tokyo in 1978. In: *Proceedings of the 15th Joint Conference on Cholera.* Bethesda, MD, US Japan Cooperative Medical Science Program, 1980:107–119.

23. Cholera surveillance. *Weekly epidemiological record*, 1980, 55(13):93–94.

24. Johnston MJ et al. Cholera in a Gulf Coast oil rig. *New England journal of medicine*, 1983, 309(9):523–526.

25. Holmberg SD et al. Foodborne transmission of cholera in Micronesian households. *Lancet*, 1984, 1(8372):325–328.

26. Goh KT et al. A common source foodborne outbreak of cholera in Singapore. *International journal of epidemiology*, 1984, 13(2):210–215.

27. Patnaik SK et al. Outbreak of cholera in Berasia Block of Bhopal District in Makhya Pradesh. *Journal of communicable diseases*, 1989, 21(2):123–128.

28. Tauxe RV et al. Epidemic cholera in Mali: high mortality and multiple routes of transmission in a famine area. *Epidemiology and infection*, 1988, 100:279–289.

29. St Louis ME et al. Epidemic cholera in West Africa: the role of food handling and high risk foods. *American journal of epidemiology*, 1990, 131(4):719–728.

30. Lowry PW et al. Cholera in Louisiana: widening spectrum of seafood vehicles. *Archives of internal medicine*, 1989, 149:2079–2084.

31. Klontz KC et al. Cholera after the consumption of raw oysters. *Annals of internal medicine*, 1987, 107:846–848.

32. Swaddiwudhipong W et al. A cholera outbreak associated with eating uncooked pork in Thailand. *Journal of diarrhoeal diseases research*, 1990, 8(3):94–96.

33. Swaddiwudhipong W, Jirakanvisun R and Rodklai A. A common source of foodborne outbreak of El Tor cholera following the consumption of uncooked beef. *Journal of the Medical Association of Thailand*, 1992, 75(7):413–417.

34. Lim-Quizon MC et al. Cholera in metropolitan Manila: foodborne transmission via street vendors. *Bulletin of the World Health Organization*, 1994, 72(5):745–749.

35. Roman et al. Cholera: New York. *Morbidity and mortality weekly report*, 1991, 40(30):516–518.

36. Weber JT et al. Epidemic cholera in Ecuador: multidrug-resistance and transmission by water and seafood. *Epidemiology and infection*, 1994, 112(1):1–11.

37. Lacey C et al. Cholera associated with imported frozen coconut milk, Maryland 1991. *Morbidity and mortality weekly report*, 40(49):844–845.

38. Cholera in clams. *New scientist*, 1991, 1786:18.

39. Koo D et al. Epidemic cholera in Guatemala, 1993: transmission of a newly introduced epidemic strain by street vendors. *Epidemiology and infection*, 1996, 116(2):121–126.

40. Cholera associated with food transported from El Salvador—Indiana, 1994. *Morbidity and mortality weekly report*, 1995, 44(20):385–386.

41. Boyce TG et al. *V. Cholerae* O139 Bengal infections among tourists to Southeast Asia: an intercontinental foodborne outbreak. *Journal of infectious diseases*, 1995, 172:1401–1404.

42. Regional information system for epidemiological surveillance of foodborne disease (SIRVE-ETA), period 1993–1994. In: *Working documents of the IX Inter-American Meeting, at the ministerial level, on animal health, Washington, DC, 25–27 April 1995.* Washington, DC, Pan American Health Organization, 1995.

43. Kam KM et al. Outbreak of *Vibrio cholerae* O1 in Hong Kong related to contaminated fish water tank. *Public health*, 1995, 109(5):389–395.

44. Levine MM et al. Volunteer studies in development of vaccines against cholera and *Escherichia coli*: a review. In: Holme T et al., eds. *Acute enteric infections in children— new prospects for treatment and prevention*. Amsterdam, Elsevier/North Holland Biochemical Press, 1974:443–459.

45. Paquet C et al. Aetiology of haemorrhagic colitis epidemic in Africa. *Lancet*, 1993, 342:175.

46. Milleliri JM et al. Toxi-infection alimentaire collective dans une structure d'acceuil pour enfants réfugiés non accompagnées de la ville de Goma, Zaïre, septembre 1994. [Collective foodborne infection in a reception centre for unaccompanied refugee children in Goma, Zaïre, September 1994.] *Cahier santé*, 1995, 5:253–257.

47. *Primera reunión de la Red Latinoamericana de Vigilancia Epidemiologica de las Enfermedades. Informe final. [First meeting of the Latin American network for the epidemiological surveillance of disease. Final report.]* Washington, DC, Pan American Health Organization, 1990.

48. Bergdoll, MS et al. Staphylococcal food poisoning in Brazil. In: *Proceedings of the 3rd World Congress on Foodborne Infections and Intoxications, Berlin, 16–19 June 1992.* Berlin, Institute of Veterinary Medicine, 1992:320–323.

49. Gao QY et al. A review of botulism in China. *Biomedical and environmental sciences,* 1990, 3:326–336.

50. Hauschild AHW. Epidemiology of foodborne botulism. In: Hauschild AWH, Dodds K, eds. *Clostridium botulinum: ecology and control in foods.* New York, Marcel Dekker Inc., 1993:68–104.

51. Wainwright RB. Hazards from Northern native foods. In: Hauschild AWH, Dodds K, eds. *Clostridium botulinum: ecology and control in foods.* New York, Marcel Dekker Inc., 1993.

52. Lund BM. Foodborne disease due to bacillus and clostridium species. *Lancet,* 1990, 336:982–986.

53. Amoebiasis. *Weekly epidemiological record,* 1997, 72(14):97–100.

54. Kefenie H, Bero G. Trichinellosis from wild boar meat in Gojjam, north west Ethiopia. *Tropical and geographical medicine,* 1992, 44(3):278–280.

55. Warren KS et al. Helminth infections. In: Jamison DT, Moseley WH, eds. *Evolving health sector priorities in the developing countries.* Washington, DC, The World Bank, 1989.

56. *Control of foodborne trematode infections. Report of a WHO Study Group.* Geneva, World Health Organization, 1995 (WHO Technical Report Series, No. 849).

57. Prevention of foodborne hepatitis A. *Weekly epidemiological record,* 1993, 68(5):25–26.

58. Public health control of hepatitis A: memorandum from a WHO meeting. *Bulletin of the World Health Organization,* 1995, 73(1):15–20.

59. Wang JY et al. Risk factor analysis of an epidemic of hepatitis A in a factory in Shanghai. *International journal of epidemiology,* 1990, 19(2):435–438.

60. Halliday ML et al. An epidemic of hepatitis A attributable to the ingestion of raw clams in Shanghai, China. *Journal of infectious disease,* 1991, 164(5):852–859.

61. Outbreak of hepatitis A—Shanghai. *Weekly epidemiological record,* 1988, 63(13):91–92.

62. Cliver DO. Virus transmission via food. *World health statistics quarterly,* 1977, 50 (1/2):90–101.

63. Djuretic T et al. General outbreaks of infectious intestinal diseases in England and Wales, 1992 to 1994. *Communicable disease report,* 1996; 6:R57–63.

64. *Advisory committee on the microbiological safety of food. Workshop on foodborne viral infections.* London, Her Majesty's Stationery Office, 1994.

65. Reid JA et al. Role of infected food handler in hotel outbreak of Norwalk virus gastroenteritis: implications for control. *Lancet*, 1988, ii:321–323.

66. Bagnis R. Ciguatera fish poisoning. In: Falconer IR, ed. *Algal toxins in seafood and drinking water*. London, Academic Press, 1993:105–115.

67. *Aquatic (marine and freshwater) biotoxins*. Geneva, World Health Organization, 1984 (Environmental health criteria, No. 37).

68. Boisier P et al. Fatal mass poisoning in Madagascar following ingestion of a shark: clinical and epidemiological aspects and isolation of toxins. *Toxicon*, 1995, 33(10):1359–1364.

69. Kao CY. Paralytic shellfish poisoning. In: Falconer IR, ed. *Algal toxins in seafood and drinking water*. San Diego, CA, Academic Press, 1993:75–86.

70. Krishnamachri KAVR et al. Hepatitis due to aflatoxicosis. An outbreak in western India. *Lancet*, 1975, May 10:1061–1063.

71. Lye MS et al. An outbreak of acute hepatic encephalopathy due to severe aflatoxicosis in Malaysia. *American journal of tropical medicine and hygiene*, 1995, 53(1):68–72.

72. Pitt JI, Hocking AD. Mycotoxigenic fungi. In: Buckle KA et al., eds. *Foodborne micro-organisms of public health significance*. Pymble (New South Wales), Australian Institute of Food Science and Technology Ltd, 1989:347–363.

73. *Mycotoxins*. Geneva, World Health Organization, 1979 (Environmental health criteria, No. 11).

74. *Selected mycotoxins: ochratoxins, tricothecenes, ergot*. Geneva, World Health Organization, 1990 (Environmental Health Criteria, No. 105).

75. Chauvin P, Dillon JC, Moren A. Épidémie d' intoxication alimentaire à l'héliotrope, Tadjikistan. [Epidemic of heliotrope infection, Tajikistan.] *Cahier santé*, 1994, 4:263–268.

76. Swaddiwuthipong W et al. Surveillance of food poisoning outbreaks in Thailand, 1981–1986. *Southeast Asian journal of tropical medicine and public health*, 1988, 19:327–331.

77. Swaddiwuthipong W et al. Foodborne disease of chemical etiology in Thailand, 1981–1986. *Southeast Asian journal of tropical medicine and public health*, 1989, 20:125–132.

78. Amin-Zaki L et al. Perinatal methylmercury poisoning in Iraq. *American journal of diseases in children*, 1976, 130:1070–1076.

79. Peters HA et al. Epidemiology of hexachlorobenzene-induced porphyria in Turkey. *Archives of neurology*, 1982, 39:744–749.

80. Motarjemi Y et al. Food safety. In: *International occupational and environmental medicine*. St. Louis, MO, Mosby, 1998:62–619.

81. Joint UNEP/FAO/WHO Food Contamination and Monitoring Programme. *Assessment of dietary intake of chemical contaminants*. Geneva, World Health Organization, 1992 (unpublished document WHO/HPP/FOS/92.F2; available on request from Programme of Food Safety, World Health Organization, 1211 Geneva 27, Switzerland).

82. *Foodborne disease in Europe: surveillance as a basis for preventive action. Report of a WHO consultation.* Copenhagen, WHO Regional Office for Europe, 1991 (unpublished document EUR/ICP/FOS 20; available on request from WHO Regional Office for Europe, 8 Scherfigsvej, DK-2100 Copenhagen Ø, Denmark).

83. Norling B. *Food poisoning in Sweden: results of a field study.* Uppsala, National Food Administration, 1994 (Report No. 41/94).

84. Hoogenboom-Verdegaal AMM et al. Bilthoven, Netherlands National Institute of Public Health and the Environment, 1990 (Report No. 148612 002).

85. Todd ECD. Preliminary estimates of costs of foodborne disease in Canada and costs to reduce salmonellosis. *Journal of food protection*, 1989, 52(8):586–594.

86. Bennett JV et al. Infections and parasitic diseases. In: Almer RW, Dull HB, eds. *Closing the gap: the burden of unnecessary illness.* New York, Oxford University Press, 1987.

87. Todd ECD. Preliminary estimates of costs of foodborne disease in the United States. *Journal of food protection*, 1989, 52(8):595–601.

88. Notermans S, Hoogenboom-Verdegaal A. Existing and emerging foodborne diseases. *International journal of food microbiology*, 1992, 15:197–205.

89. Notermans S, Van de Giessen A. Foodborne diseases in the 1980s and 1990s. *Food control*, 1993, 4(3):122–124.

90. Food Link. *Communicable disease report weekly*, 1993, 3:21 (from Public Health Laboratory Service, United Kingdom).

91. Food Link. *National food safety report 1994.* London, Food and Drink Federation, 1994.

92. Food Link. *National food safety report 1995.* London, Food and Drink Federation, 1995.

93. Hodges I. *Raw to cooked food, community awareness of safe food handling practices.* Wellington, New Zealand Department of Health, 1993.

94. Archer DL, Kvenberg JE. Incidence and cost of foodborne diarrhoeal disease in the United States. *Journal of food protection*, 1985, 48(10):887–894.

95. *Food safety from farm to table: a new strategy for the 21st century.* Washington, DC, United States Department of Agriculture, Department of Health and Human Services, and United States Environmental Protection Agency, 1997 (Internet communication of 21 February 1997 at website http://vm.cfsan.fda.gov/~dms/fs-draft.html).

96. Ten leading nationally notifiable infectious diseases, United States 1995. *Morbidity and mortality weekly report*, 1996, 45(41):883–884.

97. Fisher IST. *Salmonella enteritidis* and *S. typhimurium* in Western Europe 1993–1995: a surveillance report from Salm-net. *Europsurveillance*, 1997, 2(1):1–3.

98. Outbreaks of *Salmonella serotype enteritidis* gastroenteritis—California. *Morbidity and mortality weekly report*, 1993, R42(41):793–797.

99. Roberts D. Sources of infection: food. *Lancet*, 1990, 336:859–861.

100. *Parallel food testing in the EU. Part I: Main report, chicken.* London, International Consumer Research and Testing Ltd, 1994.

101. Jacob M. Salmonella in poultry—is there a solution? *Environmental policy and practice*, 1995, 5(2):75–80.

102. Loewenherz-Luning et al. Untersuchungen zum vorkommen von *Campylobacter jejuni* in verschiedenen Lebensmitteln tierischen Ursprungs. [Research into the appearance of *Campylobacter jejuni* in various foods of animal origin.] *Fleischwirtschaft*, 1996, 76:958–961.

103. *Salmonella in UK produced retail raw chicken.* London, Her Majesty's Stationery Office, 1996.

104. Ryan CA et al. Massive outbreak of antimicrobial-resistant salmonellosis traced to pasteurized milk. *Journal of the American Medical Association*, 1987, 258(22):3269–3274.

105. Todd ECD. Epidemiology of foodborne diseases: a worldwide review. *World health statistics quarterly*, 1997, 50(1/2):30–50.

106. *Sixth report of the WHO Surveillance Programme for Control of Foodborne Infections and Intoxications in Europe.* Berlin, Federal Institute for Health Protection of Consumers and Veterinary Medicine, 1995.

107. *Toxic oil syndrome. Current knowledge and future perspectives.* Copenhagen, WHO Regional Office for Europe, 1992 (WHO Regional Publications, European Series, No. 42).

108. *The role of food safety in health and development. Report of a joint FAO/WHO Expert Committee on Food Safety.* Geneva, World Health Organization, 1984 (WHO Technical Report Series, No. 705).

109. Hubert B. L'actualité sur les infections d'origine alimentaire en France en 1994. [The situation regarding infections originating from food in France in 1994.] *Annales de l'Institut Pasteur: Les infections d'origine alimentaire*, 1994, 5(3):163–167.

110. Vandekerckhove C, Stahl JP. La brucellose: données épidémiologiques et thérapeutiques récentes. [Brucellosis: recent epidemiological and therapeutic data.] *Médecine générale*, 1993, 7(204):47–52.

111. Young EJ. An overview of human brucellosis. *Clinical infectious diseases*, 1995, 21:283–290.

112. Morse S. Factors in emergence of infectious diseases. *Emerging infectious diseases*, 1995, 1(1):7–15.

113. Potter ME, Motarjemi Y, Kaferstein FK. Emerging foodborne disease. *World health*, 1997, 1:16–17.

114. Update on multistage outbreak of *Escherichia coli* O157:H7 infections from hamburgers, Western United States 1992–1993. *Morbidity and mortality weekly report*, 1993, 42(14):259–263.

115. Isaacson M et al. Haemorrhagic colitis epidemic in Africa. *Lancet*, 1993, 341:961.

116. Enterohaemorrhagic *E. coli* infection, Japan. *Weekly epidemiological record*, 1996, 71(35):267–268.

117. *Weekly epidemiological record*, 1997, 3(17):14–15.

118. Foodborne listeriosis. *Bulletin of the World Health Organization*, 1988, 66(4):421–428.

119. *Human listeriosis*. Geneva, World Health Organization, 1997 (unpublished document WHO/FNU/FOS/97.1; available on request from Food Safety, World Health Organization, 1211 Geneva 27, Switzerland).

120. Rocourt J. *Listeria monocytogenes*: the state of the science. *Dairy food and environmental sanitation*, 1994, 14(2):70–82.

121. Rocourt J, Bille J. Foodborne listeriosis. *World health statistics quarterly*, 1997, 50(1/2):67–73.

122. Boyce TG et al. *V. Cholerae* O139 Bengal infections among tourists to southeast Asia: an intercontinental foodborne outbreak. *Journal of infectious diseases*, 1995, 172(5):1401–1404.

123. Acute hepatitis and renal failure following ingestion of raw carp gallbladders—Maryland and Pennsylvania 1991 and 1994. *Morbidity and mortality weekly report*, August 4, 1995.

124. Käferstein FK, Motarjemi Y, Bettcher D. Control of foodborne diseases: a transnational challenge. *Emerging infectious diseases*, 1997, 3(4):503–510.

125. Hedberg CW, MacDonald KI. Changing epidemiology of foodborne disease: a Minnesota perspective. *Clinical infectious diseases*, 1994, 18:671–682.

126. Wachsmuth et al. Microbial hazards and emerging issues associated with produce. *Journal of food protection*, 1997, 60(11):1400–1408.

127. Colley DG. Widespread foodborne cyclosporiasis outbreaks present major challenges. *Emerging infectious diseases*, 1996, 2(4):354–356.

128. Hopkins RJ et al. Seroprevalence of *Helicobacter pylori* in Chile: vegetables may serve as one route of transmission. *Journal of infectious diseases*, 1993, 168:222–226.

129. *Infection with Helicobacter pylori*. Lyon, International Agency for Research on Cancer, 1994 (IARC Monographs on the Evaluation of Carcinogenic Risks to Humans, Vol. 61):177–239.

130. *Foodborne pathogens: risks and consequences*. Ames, IA, Council for Agricultural Science and Technology, 1994.

131. Brodov LE. Alimentary toxi-infections as risk factors for acute and chronic diseases (in Russian). *Terapevticheskii Arkhiv*, 1993, 65(5):77–80.

132. *Rheumatic diseases. Report of a WHO Scientific Group*. Geneva, World Health Organization, 1992 (WHO Technical Report Series, No. 816).

133. Archer DL, Young FE. Contemporary issues: diseases with a food vector. *Clinical microbiology reviews*, 1988, 1(4):377–398.

134. Watson C, Olt K. Listeria outbreak in Western Australia. *Communicable disease intelligence*, 1990, 24:9–12.

135. Desmonts G, Couvreur J. Congenital toxoplasmosis: a prospective study of 378 pregnancies. *New England journal of medicine*, 1974, 290:1110–1116.

136. Remington JS, Desmonts G. Toxoplasmosis. In: Remington JS, Klein JO, eds. *Infectious diseases of the fetus and newborn infant.* Philadelphia, Saunders, 1990:89–195.

137. Alford CA, Stagno S, Reynolds DW. Congenital toxoplasmosis: clinical laboratory and therapeutic considerations with special reference to subclinical disease. *Bulletin of the New York Academy of Medicine,* 1974, 50(2):160–181.

138. Koppe JG, Loeuer Sieger DH, de Roever-Bonnet H. Results of 20-year follow-up of congenital toxoplasmosis. *Lancet,* 1986, i:254–255.

139. *Global estimates for health situation assessment and projections.* Geneva, World Health Organization, 1990 (unpublished document WHO/HST/90.2; available on request from World Health Organization, 1211 Geneva 27, Switzerland).

140. Hlady WG, Mullen RC, Hopkins RS. *Vibrio vulnificus* from raw oysters. Leading cause of reported deaths from foodborne illness in Florida. *Journal of the Florida Medical Association,* 1993, 80(8):536–538.

141. Socket PN. The economic implications of human salmonella infection. *Journal of applied bacteriology,* 1991, 71:289–295.

142. Rocourt J. *Coût des infections bactériennes transmises par les aliments dans les pays industrialisés. [The cost of foodborne bacterial infections in industrialized countries.]* Laval, France, ASEPT Editeur, 1996.

143. Robert JA, Socket PN. The socio-economic impact of human *Salmonella enteritidis* infection. *International journal of food microbiology,* 1994, 21(1/2):117–129.

144. Fitzpatrick E. The foes in our food. *Window,* 18 August 1995.

145. Todd EC. Economic loss from foodborne disease outbreaks associated with food service establishments. *Journal of food protection,* 1985, 48(2):169–180.

146. Todd ECD. Preliminary estimates of costs of foodborne disease in Canada and costs to reduce salmonellosis. *Journal of food protection,* 1989, 52(8):586–594.

147. Todd ECD. Costs of acute bacterial foodborne disease in Canada and the United States. *International journal of food microbiology,* 1989, 9:313–326.

148. Razem D, Katusin-Razem B. The incidence and costs of foodborne diseases in Croatia. *Journal of food protection,* 1994, 57(8):746–753.

149. *Country paper on nutrition (New Zealand).* Document prepared for the FAO/WHO International Conference on Nutrition, Rome, December 1992. Wellington, Department of Health, 1992.

150. Todd ECD. Preliminary estimates of costs of foodborne disease in the United States. *Journal of food protection,* 1989, 52(8):595–601.

151. Kvenberg JE, Archer DL. Economic impact of colonization control on foodborne disease. *Food technology,* 1987, 41:77–98.

152. Archer DL, Kvenberg JE. Incidence and cost of foodborne diarrheal disease in the United States. *Journal of food protection,* 1985, 48(10):887–894.

153. Roberts T, Foegeding PM. Risk assessment for estimating the economic costs of foodborne disease caused by microorganisms. In: Caswell JA, ed. *Economics of food safety.* Amsterdam, Elsevier, 1991:103–129.

154. Garthright WE, Archer D, Kvenberg J. Estimate of incidence and costs of intestinal infectious diseases in the United States. *Public health reports*, 1988, 103(2):107–115.

155. Krug W, Rehm N. *Nutzen-kosten-analyse von Salmonellose-bekämpfung. [Cost-benefit analysis of combating salmonella.]* Schriftenreihe des Bundesministers für Jugend, Familie und Gesundheit (Document series of the Minister for Youth, Family and Health). Stuttgart, Kohlhammer, 1983.

156. Todd ECD. Social and economic impact of bacterial foodborne disease and its reduction by food irradiation and other processes. In: *IAEA/WHO/FAO International Symposium on Cost-Benefit Aspects of Food Irradiation Processing, Aix-en-Provence, France, 1–5 March 1993*. Vienna, International Atomic Energy Authority, 1993:19–49.

157. Marks S, Roberts T. *E. coli* O157:H7 ranks as fourth most costly foodborne disease. *Food review*, 1993, 16(3):51–59.

158. Roberts T, Pinner R. Economic impact of disease caused by *Listeria monocytogenes*. In: Miller AJ, Smith JL, Somkuti GA, eds. *Foodborne listeriosis*. Amsterdam, Elsevier, 1990:137–149.

159. Roberts T, Murrell KD. Economic losses caused by foodborne parasitic diseases. In: *IAEA/WHO/FAO International Symposium on Cost-Benefit Aspects of Food Irradiation Processing, Aix-en-Provence, France, 1–5 March 1993*. Vienna, International Atomic Energy Authority, 1993:51–75.

160. Velasco-Suarez M, Bravo-Bechelle MA, Quirasco F. Human cysticercosis: medical-social implications and economic impact. In: *Cysticercosis: present state of knowledge and perspectives*. New York, NY, Academic Press, 1982.

161. Loaharanu P, Sornmani S. Preliminary estimates of economic impact of liver fluke infection in Thailand and the feasibility of irradiation as a control measure. *Southeast Asian journal of tropical medicine and public health*, 1991, 22:384–390.

162. Hadler SC. Global impact of hepatitis A virus infection changing patterns. In: Hollinger FB et al., eds. *Viral hepatitis and liver disease*. Baltimore, MD, Williams & Wilkins, 1991:14–20.

163. Claeson M, Merson M. Global progress in control of diarrhoeal diseases. *Pediatric infectious disease journal*, 1990, 9:345–355.

164. Black RE et al. Longitudinal studies of infectious diseases and physical growth of children in rural Bangladesh. I: Patterns of morbidity. *American journal of epidemiology*, 1982, 115(3):305–314.

165. Black RE et al. A two year study of bacterial, viral, and parasitic agents associated with diarrhea in rural Bangladesh, *Journal of infectious diseases*, 1980, 142:660–664.

166. Forsberg BC et al. Costs of diarrhoeal diseases and the savings from a control programme in Cebu, Philippines. *Bulletin of the World Health Organization*, 1993, 71(5):579–586.

167. Motarjemi Y et al. Health and development aspects of food safety. *Archiv für Lebensmittelhygiene*, 1993, 44(2):35–41.

168. Hedberg CT, MacDonald KL, Osterholm MT. Changing epidemiology of foodborne diseases: a Minnesota perspective. *Clinical infectious diseases*, 1994, 18:671–682.

169. *Addressing emerging infectious disease threats: a preventive strategy for the United States.* Atlanta, GA, Centers for Disease Control and Prevention, 1994

170. Saadi M et al. Qualité hygiénique et nutritionelle des produits préparés et vendus par les marchands ambulants de la région de Sousse (Tunisie). [Hygienic and nutritional quality of products prepared and sold by travelling merchants in the Sousse region, Tunisia.] *Microbiologie et hygiène alimentaire*, 1996, 8(21):33–41.

171. Comité national pour l'alimentation et le développement. *Rapport du séminaire national sur l'alimentation et la nutrition, République de Côte d' Ivoire. [Report of the seminar on food and nutrition, Republic of Ivory Coast.]* Document prepared for the FAO/WHO International Conference on Nutrition, Rome. December 1992.

172. Ries AA et al. Cholera in Piura, Peru: a modern urban epidemic. *Journal of infectious diseases*, 1992, 166:1429–1433.

173. Compton SJ et al. Trichinosis with ventilatory failure and persistent myocarditis. *Clinical infectious diseases*, 1993, 16:500–504.

174. Sherbeeny MR, Saddik MF, Bryan FL. Microbiological profiles of foods served by street vendors in Egypt. *International journal of food microbiology*, 1985, 2:355–364.

175. *Report on street-vended and weaning foods in Yangon, Myanmar.* Geneva, World Health Organization, 1995 (unpublished document; available on request from Food Safety, World Health Organization, 1211 Geneva 27, Switzerland).

176. Howie JW. Typhoid in Aberdeen 1964. *Journal of applied bacteriology*, 1968, 31:171–178.

177. Kapperud G et al. Outbreak of *Shigella sonnei* infection traced to imported iceberg lettuce. *Journal of clinical microbiology*, 1995, 33(3):609–614.

178. *International tourism overview. A special report of the World Tourism Organization.* Barcelona, World Tourism Organization, 1996.

179. Cossar JH, Reid D. Health hazards of international travel. *World health statistics quarterly*, 1989, 42:61–69.

180. Steffen R, Lobel HO. Travel medicine. In: Cook GC, ed. *Manson's tropical diseases*, 20th ed. London, WB Saunders, 1996.

181. Cartwright RY, Chahed M. Foodborne diseases in travellers. *World health statistics quarterly*, 1997, 50(1/2):102–110.

182. Kozicki M, Steffen R, Schär M. Boil it, cook it, peel it or forget it: does this rule prevent travellers' diarrhoea? *International journal of epidemiology*, 1985 14(1):169–172.

183. Hirn J et al. Long-term experience with competitive exclusion and salmonellas in Finland. *International journal of food microbiology*, 1992, 15(3–4):281–285.

184. Parsonnet J et al. *Shigella dysenteriae* Type 1: infections in US travellers to Mexico. *Lancet*, 1989, September 2:543–545.

185. Mathieu JJ et al. Typhoid fever in New York City, 1980 through 1990. *Archives of internal medicine*, 1994, 154(15):1713–1718.

186. Yew FS, Goh KT, Lim YS. Epidemic of typhoid fever in Singapore. *Epidemiology and infection*, 1993, 110(1):63–70.

187. Bryan FL. Risks of practices, procedures and processes that lead to outbreaks of foodborne diseases. *Journal of food protection*, 1988, 51(8):663–673.

188. Bean NH, Griffin PM. Foodborne disease outbreaks in the United States, 1973–1987: pathogens, vehicles and trends. *Journal of food protection*, 1990, 53(9):804–817.

189. Beckers HJ. Incidence of foodborne diseases in the Netherlands: annual summary, 1980. *Journal of food protection*, 1985, 48(2):181–187.

190. Alkanahl HA, Gasim Z. Foodborne disease incidents in the Eastern Province of Saudi Arabia—a five year summary, 1982–1986. *Journal of food protection*, 1993, 55(1):84–87.

191. Oldfield III EC, Wallace MR. Endemic infectious disease of the Middle East. *Review of infectious diseases*, 1991, 13(Suppl 3):S199–S217.

192. Merlin M et al. Toxi-infections alimentaires collectives dans les armées. Evolution des tendances sur 5 ans. [Collective foodborne infections in armies. Evolution of trends over 5 years.] *Médecine et armées*, 1990, 18(5):327–329.

193. Gastroenteritis aboard planes. *Morbidity and mortality weekly report*, 1971, 20(8):149.

194. Shigellosis related to airline meal—northeastern United States. *Morbidity and mortality weekly report*, 1971, 20:397, 402.

195. Peffers ASR et al. *Vibrio parahaemolyticus* gastroenteritis and international travel. *Lancet*, 1973, i:143–145.

196. Dakin WPH et al. Gastroenteritis due to non-agglutinable (non-cholera) vibrios. *Medical journal of Australia*, 1974, 2:487–490.

197. Tauxe RV et al. Salmonellosis outbreak on transatlantic flights. Foodborne illness on aircraft: 1947–1984. *American journal of epidemiology*, 1987, 125(1):150–157.

198. Eisenberg MS et al. Staphylococcal food poisoning aboard a commercial aircraft. *Lancet*, 1975, 2:595–599.

199. Foodborne *Salmonella* infections contracted on aircraft. *Weekly epidemiological record*, 1976, 51:265–266.

200. Outbreak of staphylococcal food poisoning aboard an aircraft. *Morbidity and mortality weekly report*, 1976, 25:317–318.

201. Burselm CD, Kelly M, Preston FS. Food poisoning—a major threat to airline operations. *Journal of the Society of Occupational Medicine*, 1990, 40:97–100.

202. Hatakka M. *Salmonella* outbreak among railway and airline passengers. *Acta veterinaria Scandinavica*, 1992, 33:253–260.

203. Hedberg CW et al. An international foodborne outbreak of shigellosis associated with a commercial airline. *Journal of the American Medical Association*, 1992, 268(22):3208–3212.

204. Jahkola M. *Salmonella enteritidis* outbreak traced to airline food. *WHO Surveillance Programme for Control of Foodborne Infections and Intoxications in Europe, newsletter* 22:3. Berlin, Institute of Veterinary Medicine, 1989.

205. Sockett P, Ries A, Wieneke AA. Food poisoning associated with in-flight meals. *Communicable disease report*, 1993, 3(7):R103–R104.

206. Lester R et al. Air travel associated gastroenteritis. *Communicable diseases intelligence*, 1991, 15(17):292–293.

207. Eberhart-Philips J et al. An outbreak of cholera from food served on an international aircraft. *Epidemiology and infection*, 1996, 116:9–13.

208. *Rapport du seminaire national sur l'alimentation et la nutrition, Abidjan, Côte d'Ivoire, du 9 au 12 mars, 1992. [Report of a national seminar on food and nutrition, Abidjan, Côte d'Ivoire, 9–12 March 1992.]* Abidjan, National Committee for Food and Development, 1992.

209. Rampal L. A food poisoning outbreak due to *Staphylococcus aureus*, Kapar, Malaysia. *Medical journal for Malaysia*, 1983, 38(4):294–298.

210. Belongia EA et al. An outbreak of *Escherichia coli* O157:H7 associated with consumption of precooked meat patties. *Journal of infectious diseases*, 1991, 164:338–343.

211. Kulshrestha SB et al. Enterotoxigenic *Eschericha coli* from an outbreak with cholerogenic syndromes of gastroenteritis. *Journal of communicable diseases*, 1989, 21(4):313–317.

212. Weaver LT et al. *Salmonella typhi* infection associated with a school feeding programme. *Journal of tropical pediatrics*, 1989, 35:331–333.

213. Richard MS et al. Investigation of a staphylococcal food poisoning outbreak in a centralized lunch program. *Public health reports*, 1993, 108(6):765–771.

214. Blostein J. An outbreak of *Salmonella javiana* associated with consumption of water melon. *Journal of environmental health*, 1993, 56(1):29–31.

215. Oishi I et al. A large outbreak of acute gastroenteritidis associated with astrovirus among students and teachers in Osaka, Japan. *Journal of infectious diseases*, 1994, 170:439–443.

216. Al-Zubaidy AA, El Bushra HE, Mawlawi MY. An outbreak of typhoid fever among children who attended a pot-luck dinner at Al-Mudhnab, Saudi Arabia. *East African medical journal*, 1995, 72(6):373–375.

217. Solodovinikov IUP et al. Food poisoning in a boarding school. *Zhurnal mikrobiologii, epidemiologii i immunobiologii*, 1996, 4:121.

218. Solodovinikov IUP, Serzhenko SV, Pozdeeva LI. An outbreak of food poisoning at a children's rest base. *Zhurnal mikrobiologii, epidemiologii i immunobiologii*, 1996, 4(4):120–121.

219. Khodr M et al. *Bacillus cereus* food poisoning associated with fried rice at two day care centres—Virginia 1993. *Morbidity and mortality weekly report*, 1994, 27(14):1074.

220. Toyokawa Y et al. Large outbreak of *Yersinia pseudotuberculosis* serotype 5a infection at Noheji-machi in Aomori prefecture. *Kansenshogaku-zasshi*, 1993, 67(1):36–44.

221. Stuart J et al. Outbreak of campylobacter enteritidis in a residential school associated with bird pecked bottle tops. *Communicable disease report review*, 1997, 7(3):R38–R40.

222. Gelletie R et al. Cryptosporidiosis associated with school milk. *Lancet*, 1997, 350:1005–1006.

223. Adams RM. Let's do lunch: food poisoning at school. *Pediatric infectious diseases journal*, 1996, 15(3):274–276.

224. Outbreak among school children in Sakai city. *Weekly epidemiological record*, 1996, 35:267–268.

225. *Food safety matters*. ICD/SEAMEO Food safety gazette for nutritionists, July–September 1997, supplement No. 7.

226. *Vibrio parahaemolyticus. Japan, 1987–1993*. Tokyo, Infectious Agents Surveillance Center, 1994.

227. Abdusalam M et al. Food related behaviour. In: Hamburg D, Sartorius N, eds. *Health and behaviour: selected perspectives*. Cambridge, Cambridge University Press, 1989:45–64.

228. *Guidlelines for strengthening a national food safety programme*. Geneva, World Health Organization, 1996 (unpublished document WHO/FUN/FOS/96.2; available on request from Food Safety, World Health Organization, 1211 Geneva 27, Switzerland).

229. *Management of food control programmes*. Rome, Food and Agriculture Organization of the United Nations, 1989.

230. Motarjemi Y et al. Importance of HACCP for public health and development; the role of the World Health Organization. *Food control*, 1996, 7(2):77–85.

CHAPTER 2

Why health education in food safety?

The prevention of foodborne diseases requires a combined regulatory and educational approach. This chapter explains why the education of food handlers and consumers is particularly important.

Food preparation: a critical stage in the food chain

The food chain varies in length and complexity according to the degree of urbanization or industrialization. It may include the following stages (Fig. 8):

— primary production (agriculture, animal husbandry and fishery involving farmers and fishermen);
— processing and manufacturing by large or cottage (artisanal) industries;
— transport, storage and distribution involving retailers and supermarkets;
— preparation for consumption by food service and catering establishments, street food vendors, and domestic food handlers preparing the family food.

In rural areas, some or all of the stages of the food chain may be carried out at household or artisanal level (e.g. subsistence farmers may live on foods that are produced, processed and prepared in their own households).

The prevention of foodborne diseases requires that contamination be prevented or controlled at all stages of the food chain from production to consumption. However, measures implemented at the earlier stages of the food chain will be effective only if measures are also applied at later stages, particularly when food is being prepared for consumption.

The strategy for preventing foodborne illnesses can be described in terms of three lines of defence—improvement of the hygienic quality of raw foodstuffs in agriculture and aquaculture, application of food processing technologies that control contaminants, and education of consumers and food handlers.

Experience has shown that, despite all efforts in agriculture, the production of food of animal origin free from pathogens (first line of defence) is not yet possible, and a large proportion of foodstuffs reaching consumers is contaminated (*1, 2*). Contamination of foodstuffs is sometimes unavoidable as some organisms belong to the natural flora of the human environment. Toxins may also be naturally present in foods. Sometimes, the natural components of food have anti-nutritional consequences and need to be denatured or inhibited during food preparation (trypsin inhibitors, lectins). In such cases, hazards may be present in foods regardless of agricultural or aquacultural practices.

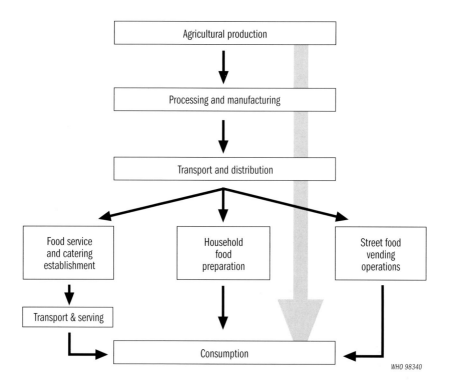

Fig. 8. A model food chain

The second line of defence (i.e. the application of food processing technologies to eliminate or reduce pathogens or contaminants) is also not sufficient by itself to ensure food safety. For economic or other reasons, processing technologies are not available for the treatment of all foods or for the elimination of all pathogens. Foods can be recontaminated after processing, particularly during food preparation by food handlers who themselves may be carriers of pathogens.

Thus, the third line of defence—the education of food handlers and consumers in the hygienic handling of food—is crucial in preventing foodborne illnesses and will be effective even when the other two defences fail. As the preparation of food for consumption is at the end of the food chain, it is a critical stage. Any contamination, whether introduced earlier or resulting from handling during preparation, which is not controlled at this stage will have a direct negative bearing on the health of the consumer.

Education of the public and of domestic and professional food handlers in safe food preparation is essential to ensure that:

— food is not contaminated by them;

49

— contaminants that may be present in foodstuffs are eliminated or reduced to safe levels;
— the growth of microorganisms to disease-causing levels, or the production of toxin, is prevented;
— contaminated food which cannot be rendered safe is avoided.

Routine food processing

A substantial amount of food handling and processing occurs in homes, in food service and catering establishments, or in street food vending operations. In rural areas and in developing countries, where industrially processed food is not readily available or affordable, food is processed to a greater extent at household level. Sometimes the whole food chain from farming to consumption occurs at the home. The efforts of environmental movements in industrialized countries have led some consumers to become increasingly interested in home-processed food.

Whenever food is processed in industry, health authorities can exert some control over the quality and safety of the product through legislation and inspection. In addition, the reputation and commercial interests of the company are often incentive enough to implement a system of self-control. Many large-scale food companies have access to laboratories and qualified scientists to ensure the safety of the food they produce.

Formal/official control (inspection and analysis of food samples) is, however, not possible at household level and has been shown to have limitations in food service and catering establishments or street food operations. Yet the kind of processing and manufacturing that takes place at industrial level may also take place in households or food service and catering establishments. Thus the main way to control the safety of food prepared in households and food service establishments is to provide food handlers and consumers with the know-how to handle food safely. In other words, the control must be exercised by the food handlers themselves and, in order to do this, they must be informed, educated and, in the case of professional food handlers, properly trained.

It should be remembered that many food technologies have been developed on the basis of trial and error in homes or small industries. Scientists understand how food technologies work and what factors determine the safety of a food product. However, because of lack of communication, this knowledge has remained with scientists and has not always been properly communicated to the public. Many consumers and food handlers prepare foods using knowhow that they or previous generations have acquired empirically. In the absence of thorough understanding of the consequences of their actions, such know-how does not always guarantee the safety of food in all situations. Whenever the conditions for food preparation change (e.g. the quantity and number of dishes to be prepared increases, the ambient temperature goes up, or a new pathogen is present in the raw foodstuff), the scene is set for an outbreak. It has been noted that outbreaks commonly occur during holidays and banquets when food is prepared in large quantities and often in advance. During the summer months, the incidence of foodborne diseases increases due partly to a rise in ambient temperatures that favours bacterial growth.

The problem of the disease called konzo in Africa is an example of how a change in the socioeconomic setting can result in a food safety problem. In this case the problem arose because of lack of understanding of food handlers of the significance of their actions when processing cassava. Epidemics of konzo, a form of myelopathy characterized by an abrupt onset of spastic paraparesis, have been known to occur in sub-Saharan Africa. Studies of outbreaks in the Bandundu region of the Democratic Republic of the Congo have attributed these outbreaks to exposure to cyanide from the consumption of inadequately processed cassava. Cassava contains natural cyanogens, and the traditional processing in Africa includes a period of soaking during which the cyanogens are removed. In the mid 1970s a new road to the capital was constructed. This increased the demand for cash crops. To respond to the higher demand, the women who processed the cassava reduced the soaking time from three days to one. This resulted in a higher content of cyanogen, which led to outbreaks of konzo in the dry season since during this period the diet lacks supplementary foods with the sulfur-containing amino acids that are essential for cyanide detoxification (*3*).

The managers of food service establishments, as well as street food vendors, are often persons with no specific know-how in food safety. They prepare food on the basis of the knowledge they have acquired from the preparation of food at home, unaware that rules for the safe preparation of food in large quantities differ from those for preparing family food. For instance, large quantities of food require a longer time to cool to safe temperatures, unless care is taken to divide the large amounts into smaller batches or the kitchen is equipped with a refrigerator with an air circulation (convection) system which increases the rate of heat transfer. Also, the risk of cross-contamination is much higher in food service establishments where numerous dishes are prepared simultaneously, often in a limited space. In over-full refrigerators, foods may also take longer to cool to safe temperatures. The same risks are present when food is prepared for banquets or for mass feeding in refugee camps. In all these circumstances, only a properly trained or educated food handler can ensure that appropriate safety precautions are taken while the food is being prepared.

Epidemiological studies worldwide show that, in the majority of cases, outbreaks of foodborne diseases are due to the incorrect handling of food by food handlers in homes, food service and catering establishments or street food vending operations—i.e. during the final stage of food preparation (Table 12).

Table 12. Percentage of factors that contributed to the occurrence of outbreaks of foodborne diseases (a) for selected foodborne diseases and (b) for different locations where food is prepared (Source: 4)

(a) Percentage of factors that contributed to the occurrence of outbreaks of certain foodborne disease in England and Wales (E/W) and the USA[a]

Factors	Salmonellosis		Staphylococcal enterotoxicosis		Clostridium perfringens gastro-enteritis		Bacillus cereus gastro-enteritis	Botulism	Shigellosis	Typhoid fever	Vibrio parahaemolyticus gastro-enteritis
	USA (238)	E/W (396)	USA (214)	E/W (133)	USA (93)	E/W (387)	E/W (53)	USA (85)	USA (27)	(USA) (14)	USA (12)
Factors affecting growth of pathogens											
Preparation too far in advance	21[b]	49	47	56	63	92	94		26		67
Foods left at room temperature	47	29	78	41	76	54	60	13	56	7	
Foods cooled in large pots		18		8		61	30				
Improper warm-holding	14	2	18		46	11	15	2		7	
Improper thawing		11				6					
Extra-large quantities prepared	–[c]	3		2	–	4					
Faulty fermentation	1	–		–		–	–	9			

Factor										
Factors affecting survival of pathogens										
Inadequate thermal processing or cooking	21	23	3	1	9[d]	16[d]	2	80		
Inadequate reheating	13	12	7[e]	3[e]	45	56	55	2	7	
Factors affecting contamination										
Contaminated raw food or ingredient	32	9					2			42
Infected person	13	2	53	33					89	79
Cross-contamination	21	14	3	2	2	1				33
Inadequate cleaning of equipment	15	—	9	—	1	—	—	—	—	
Unsafe source	1	—	—	—	—	—	—	—	—	14
Contaminated water (sea)	—	—	—	—	—	—	—	—	—	8

[a] Number of outbreaks analysed in parenthesis. More than one factor was usually considered responsible for an outbreak.

[b] Includes preparation 1 day or more in advance (USA); half a day in advance (E/W); and use of leftovers.

[c] — = data not summarized.

[d] Spores of *C. perfringens* not always killed by cooking.

[e] Reheating not likely to destroy enterotoxin.

Table 12. *Continued*

(b) Percentage of factors that contributed to the occurrence of outbreaks of foodborne diseases in Canada, England and Wales, and the USA[a]

Factors	USA, 1973–76			USA, 1961–76 (1152 outbreaks)	England and Wales, 1970–79 (1044 outbreaks)	Canada, 1973–77 (805 outbreaks)
	Food-service establishments (235 outbreaks)	Homes (122 outbreaks)	Food-processing establishments (32 outbreaks)			
Factors affecting growth of pathogens						
Preparation too far in advance	36	11	100[b]	21[b]	66	8
Foods left at room temperature	63	30	16	31	40	26
Foods cooled in large pots				15	32	
Improper warm-holding	26	6	0	16	6	3
Improper thawing	1	0	0	<1	6	–
Extra-large quantities prepared	–[c]	–	–	–	3	–
Factors affecting survival of pathogens						
Inadequate thermal processing or cooking	5	21	25	16	15	24
Inadequate reheating	25	5	0	12	29	–

Factors affecting contamination

Contaminated raw ingredient	2	22	25	11	4	3
Infected person	26	8	9	20	5	6
Cross-contamination	6	2	0	7	6	
Inadequate cleaning of equipment	9	1	6	7	–	
Food from unsafe source	1	11	0	5	–	
Contaminated canned food	0	1	–	–	4	7
Contaminated processed food (not canned)	0	6	22	–	19	–
Toxic containers	4	1	0	2	–	
Toxic plants mistaken for edible foods	0	13	0	–	–	3
Incidental additives	2	0	6	<1	–	
Intentional additives	1	0	3	2	–	
Inadequate sanitation	–	–	–	–	–	3
Poor handling practices	–	–	–	–	–	3

[a] In the reports from the USA and England and Wales more than one factor was usually considered to be responsible for an outbreak. For Canada only the factor regarded as the most important in each outbreak was recorded; 14% of outbreaks were due to factors not listed here.

[b] All foods prepared days before use.

[c] = data not summarized.

55

Experience in industrialized and developing countries

Many countries, particularly industrialized ones, have an extensive food control infrastructure, including food legislation that is updated regularly and effective enforcement mechanisms. Experience from these countries shows that a comprehensive and well-funded regulatory system alone cannot prevent foodborne disease. The high and increasing incidence of foodborne disease in industrialized countries is evidence of this.

On the other hand, wherever regulatory and educational measures have been combined they have proven to be effective in reducing foodborne disease. A good example is action taken in the United Kingdom and USA to prevent listeriosis. Combined regulatory and educational measures have been successful in reducing the incidence of this disease significantly (see page 65) (5, 6).

Unfortunately, examples of a combined regulatory and educational approach are scarce. Many countries still rely solely on a regulatory approach for the prevention of foodborne diseases. In settings where most food is processed and prepared at home, such as in some developing countries or in the case of people living on subsistence farming, a regulatory approach to food safety can be of only limited value. Thus, education of public, and particularly of domestic food handlers, takes on even greater importance for the prevention of foodborne diseases.

In developing countries, most efforts to prevent diarrhoeal disease have focused on improving the water supply and sanitation. Regrettably, in many instances the provision of safe water and sanitation has been an end in itself and has not been combined with an effective educational programme on the hygienic handling of food including water. A critical review of the impact of improved water supplies and excreta disposal facilities in the control of diarrhoeal diseases among young children has shown that, even under the most favourable conditions, the rate of morbidity was reduced by only 27% (7). While such measures are unquestionably essential to food safety and health, their efficiency in reducing diarrhoeal diseases would be much enhanced if they were combined with a food hygiene education programme that included education in the safe use and storage of water and efficient handwashing prior to food preparation. Indeed, experience from industrialized countries where a safe water supply and excreta disposal facilities are available indicates that the provision of a safe water supply and sanitation *per se* is not sufficient to prevent diarrhoeal diseases, since the incidence of many of these diseases has continued to increase (8). In many developing countries, great progress has been made in the provision of safe water and today a great percentage of the population benefit from this. Nevertheless, diarrhoeal diseases in infants and children remain a major cause of morbidity and mortality in these countries.

Worldwide, mortality from infant diarrhoea in developing countries has decreased. However, this decrease is due mainly to the improved clinical management of cases rather than to the effectiveness of prevention measures. Children saved by oral rehydration salts (ORS) may continue to suffer from diarrhoeal diseases and associated malnutrition, and may become weaker and weaker until they die from another kind of infection.

With regard to industrialized countries it should be realized that, with increased international travel and trade, national regulatory measures will not be sufficient to protect populations from foodborne diseases. In Sweden, where a comprehensive programme aiming at the elimination of salmonella-contaminated poultry is being implemented, the incidence of salmonellosis is nevertheless very high and comparable to that in other European countries. One of the reasons for this is that 80–90% of cases of salmonellosis are travel-related. Improved education of travellers may thus decrease the incidence of salmonellosis.

Shared responsibility

Food safety means that when food is consumed it does not contain contaminants at levels which cause harm. All persons, whether they prepare food or only consume it, are part of the food chain. As such they share responsibility with government and the food industry in ensuring the safety of food. This concept of shared responsibility is illustrated in Fig. 9.

People can take a responsibility for food safety only if they receive professional advice on the risks that certain foods or practices pose to their health. They need also to be guided in their choice of food. For instance, consumers need to be informed—and constantly reminded—of the risk of certain raw foodstuffs, particularly those of animal origin. Incidences of foodborne disease occur repeatedly due to the consumption of raw meat, raw milk and raw seafood. Many cases of milkborne diseases have occurred due to the consumption of raw milk during visits by schoolchildren to farms. Unfortunately, in some industrialized countries, the trend to consuming so-called "health foods" has induced many persons to consume raw milk without being aware of the risks they take.

In cases where a new pathogen is emerging, or a pre-existing pathogen is adopting new epidemiological features (e.g. *Salmonella enteritidis* contaminating the content of eggs), the general public needs to be advised about the new pathogen, its mode of transmission and necessary control measures so that they can take steps to protect themselves.

International trade in food has been facilitated by the development of food technologies and transportation and by international travel and migration. However, as a result of this international trade, the diet of a population may

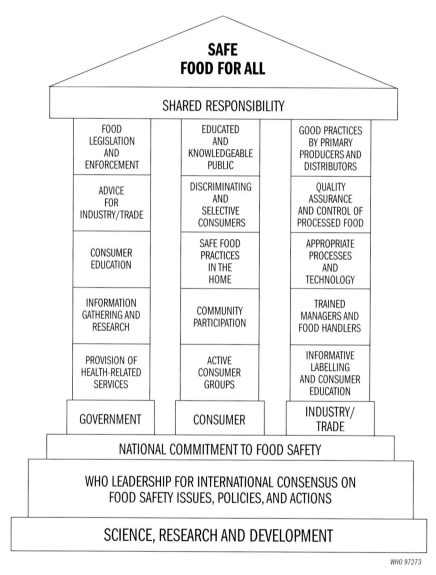

Fig. 9. The concept of shared responsibility

change. People may consume foodstuffs that are strange to them or may adopt new ways of preparing food. As each food and food preparation practice has its own characteristics and potential hazards, it is imperative to educate consumers about hazards that may be introduced by the new foods or methods of preparation. For instance, the introduction to North America of the Japanese tradition of eating raw fish has led to many cases of anisakiasis there.

People have the right to be informed of the hazards of new foodstuffs, food preparation practices or technologies. They need to be educated about how to keep food safe. Similarly, travellers should be informed of the risks in the places they will visit. It is only an educated and informed consumer who can share responsibility with government and industry in food safety (see also Box 4).

Box 4. Consumer rights in the USA

The four main consumer rights, emphasized by former US President J. F. Kennedy in his message on consumer rights in March 1962 were (9):

– the right to safety

– the right to be informed

– the right to choose

– the right to be heard.

High-risk groups

Certain people are subject to greater risk of contracting foodborne infections and intoxications than others. Two high-risk groups can be distinguished—travellers because they are more likely to be exposed to contaminated food, and vulnerable people because they are more susceptible. Travellers are at higher risk because they lack immunity to the microbiological flora of the countries they visit, and they have a higher degree of exposure to pathogens because they are usually obliged to eat in food service establishments or purchase food from street food vendors. Vulnerable persons are those who, for physiological or other reasons, are more susceptible to foodborne infections. They include infants and children, the elderly, pregnant women, persons who are undernourished, those with underlying illness (e.g. liver disease, diabetes), and those who are immunocompromised due either to an infection (e.g. AIDS) or to medical treatment (e.g. cancer patients). Vulnerable groups represent an important segment of the population. In the USA it has been estimated that they make up 20% of the population and this percentage is expected to increase significantly by the beginning of the next century because of increases in life expectancy and the number of immunocompromised persons (*10*).

Vulnerable persons are not only at higher risk of contracting a foodborne illness but may also suffer more severely. For example, it has been demonstrated that the fatality rate of elderly persons from salmonellosis is 10 times higher than that of the rest of the population (*11*). Persons with liver disease run a risk of infection with *Vibrio vulnificus* that is 80 times greater than that of others, and a risk of death that is 200 times greater (*12*). More than half of documented deaths from gastroenteritis and hepatitis A occur in elderly persons in developing countries (*10*).

According to some studies, individuals (including infants) with HIV infection are more likely to suffer from diarrhoea than those not infected. Diarrhoea also leads to more rapid progression of HIV. Diarrhoea due to intestinal infection is observed in 30–60% of HIV cases and is even considered as one of the manifestations of HIV (*13, 14*).

In view of the effect of foodborne pathogens on the health of these groups, it is imperative to inform them of the increased risk they run from contaminated food and to advise them of the precautions they can take to protect themselves.

It is important to note that absolute safety is not attainable. Foods that are regarded as safe for the general population may be unsafe for individuals who have food intolerance or allergies, lack immunity or have underlying health conditions that make them vulnerable (see also Box 5). These persons should be notified of the increased risks that certain foods may pose to them. The importance of this kind of advice is well recognized in connection with allergies; regulatory agencies in many countries require the labelling of additives or substances which may be allergenic to some individuals. It is equally important to advise high-risk groups about food safety concerns that are important to their health. Managers of food service establishments should also be advised to not recommend foods which may entail a health risk for certain groups (e.g. raw or undercooked eggs, foods containing raw eggs, raw meat).

Box 5. Food allergies (*15–18*)

In addition to foodborne diseases, foods may cause different types of nontoxic adverse reactions such as food allergies. A food allergy is an adverse reaction to an otherwise harmless food or food component that involves the body's immune system in the production of antigen-specific immunoglobulin E to specific substances in foods.

Surveys suggest that one-third of all adults believe that they have at one time or another had food allergies. Yet true food allergy is estimated to affect less than 1–2% of the population. Children are at greater risk with up to 5% of infants having food allergies which they often outgrow. Allergic reactions can occur to virtually any food, though most reactions are caused by a limited number of foods. Some of the most common allergenic foods are eggs, milk, fish, crustacea, peanuts, soybeans, wheat and tree nuts.

In most cases, food allergies are an inconvenience that results in unpleasant symptoms. However, for some individuals who are highly sensitive to particular foods (e.g. peanuts) the results can be life-threatening. Allergic reactions usually begin within a few minutes to a few hours after eating the allergenic food. Very sensitive persons may experience an allergic reaction even from exposure to trace quantities of the offending food. The symptoms include anaphylaxis and symptoms from the skin (e.g. angiooedema, urticaria, eczema, erythema), respiratory organs (rhinitis, sneezing, asthma) and gastrointestinal tract (nausea, vomiting, diarrhoea, colic, abdominal pain).

It is important that food handlers working in food service establishments, including cooks and waiters, are fully aware of the importance of food allergies for some persons, even if it concerns only a small number of the population. Food handlers should carefully read the documentation on the processed or semi-processed foods that they use, and at all times they should be aware of the content of the food they serve to customers.

Individuals allergic to specific foods should avoid them. Careful reading of food labels is advised.

New food technologies

Food science and technology are evolving rapidly. Consumers are faced with the products of new technologies (e.g. irradiated and vacuum-packed food products) or are using new technologies at homes (e.g. freezing and microwave heating). In either case, consumers need to be informed of safety concerns regarding the new technologies. A lack of understanding of new technologies may lead either to their rejection or to their incorrect use.

For instance, lack of understanding and misuse of microwave heating has resulted in a variety of health problems. Incidents have been reported of eggs exploding during microwave cooking and causing eye injury, or of children receiving burns and scalds from food prepared by microwave (*19–21*). Undercooking of foods and survival of pathogens due to non-uniform distribution of heat in food ("cold spots") have been reported (*22–25*). Outbreaks of foodborne disease associated with microwave cooking have also been reported (*26, 27*). There have been also cases of babies being scalded because bottles of infant formula were warmed in a microwave oven in such a way that the content was boiling but the container was still cold.

Another result of new technology is the production of conventional foods with fewer calories—so-called "light foods". Consumers do not always realize that such foods may require different storage or handling. Vacuum packaging and its potential in preserving foods is also not well understood so there is risk in incorrect handling such products in the home (*28*).

People's fears of unfamiliar food technologies may also lead them to reject technologies that may be beneficial to their health. One example is food irradiation which has been shown to be a powerful tool in eliminating many pathogens from food.

The experts	The public
1. Microbial safety	1. Pesticides
2. Over/undernutrition	2. New food chemicals
3. Non-microbial safety	3. Additives
a. contaminants	4. Fat and cholesterol
b. natural toxins	5. Microbial spoilage
c. agriculture chemicals	6. Junk foods

WHO 98343

Fig. 10. How expert and public concerns about food safety differ (Source: Reproduced with permission from *29*)

Awareness and risk perception

Experts and the general public often differ in their perceptions of risk. While experts judge hazards on the basis of the scientific process of risk assessment, the general public base their judgement on criteria that are influenced by factors other than science (such as traditional beliefs, culture, mass media, personal experience) (*29*). Fig. 10 represents the difference in expert and public perception of hazards in the USA a few years ago. The figure is still representative of the situation in many countries (*30*).

Members of the public, and sometimes even policy-makers and public health authorities, have subjective or inaccurate perceptions of the risks associated with food. Not infrequently they may overlook the imminent food safety problems. In industrialized countries, although most cases of foodborne diseases are of microbial origin and may stem from mishandling of food during its preparation, the concern of consumers has centred on chemicals such as pesticides and food additives.

Many consumers are turning to so-called "health foods" in the hope of avoiding chemicals. They ignore the fact that food is itself a mixture of chemical substances and that many of the substances they fear may occur naturally in food. In this regard, if one does not properly balance the risks and benefits of "health foods" one may expose oneself to even greater health hazards. The perception that unprocessed foods are of a higher nutritional quality has led some consumers to drink raw milk, thus exposing themselves to milkborne pathogens such as *Campylobacter, Salmonella, E. coli* O157, *Cryptosporidium*.

Some nutritional scientists have been instrumental in promoting such trends by recommending certain dietary practices without considering the food safety consequences. For example, to avoid the formation of mutagenic compounds during food preparation (e.g. during grilling and frying of protein-rich foods) people have been advised to avoid heating for long periods of time. Fears of potential mutagenic compounds have influenced some consumers to undercook meat, despite the fact that undercooked meat may be a more immediate and much greater health risk.

Honey is known to have many nutritional qualities and many parents, in the belief of giving nutritious food to their infants, may expose them to the risk of infant botulism. Honey may contain *Clostridium botulinum.* Although ingestion of this microorganism does not present a health risk in adults, it may cause infant botulism.

Another common misperception relates to the problem of diarrhoeal diseases in developing countries. In many societies, diarrhoea is not seen as a symptom of a disease with severe health consequence but is considered a "natural" health problem (see also Box 6). People may also ignore the role of food and food-handling in the transmission of diarrhoeal diseases, particularly infant diarrhoea, and may attribute it to other factors such as indigestion, teething, eating "hot foods", the quality of breast milk, or sorcery. In a community-based study of the etiology of diarrhoea in Papua New Guinea, children whose mothers did not perceive babies' faeces to be contaminated and therefore important in causing diarrhoea had a 7.4 times greater risk of having diarrhoea than children whose mothers recognized this importance. The risk of contamination of food was 6.8 times greater for those children whose mothers did not recognize the importance of this route (*33*). A survey of knowledge among mothers in the rural communities of two villages in the Sudan (87 literate and 152 illiterate mothers) showed that most attributed di-

---

Box 6. Causes of diarrhoea as perceived in different cultures (*32*)

1. Foods that are fatty, not cooked adequately or heavy.

2. Imbalance of heat and cold associated with food, exposure to draughts or seasonal changes.

3. Normal or poor quality of breast milk.

4. Physical factors such as a fall or poor care of the child.

5. Supernatural causes, including possession, sorcery or the evil eye.

6. Pollution from exposure to or inauspicious contact with ritually impure persons or things.

7. Moral misbehaviour, including the deeds of the sick person or a sick child's parents, especially promiscuous sex and sexual intercourse or pregnancy while breast-feeding.

8. Natural consequences of developmental milestones, especially teething, crawling and walking.

9. Infection which may be associated with hygiene and sanitation (but which may be thought to be due to pollution).

---

arrhoea in their children to teething (*34*). Even in industrialized countries, many people do not appreciate the relationship between bacteria and the human and animal body and are unaware that the body is host to both non-pathogenic and pathogenic bacteria which can pass into food (*35*).

Most cultures define faeces as dirty but they are not always perceived as a cause of disease. There is a widespread belief that the faeces of infants and small children are harmless. This is even true in industrialized countries. Some mothers in the United States have been observed not to wash their hands after changing diapers (*36*). In general, the perception of cleanliness is not always based on germ theory. In Bangladesh, for instance, cleanliness in terms of personal hygiene is viewed in the larger socioreligious context of purity and impurity. Washing oneself serves both physical and spiritual needs and is performed according to defined patterns that may not effectively prevent contamination of food by food handlers. Soap is generally considered a cosmetic rather than an agent for the removal of microorganisms (*37*).

Even if people have information, they may be subjective or unrealistic about it (*38*). They may be overoptimistic about falling ill. It is often observed that, despite the knowledge of the risk of eating raw foods of animal origin or raw seafood, people nevertheless do so because of ingrained cultural habits or because of a resistance to giving up something they see as pleasurable.

Consumers often judge the safety of a food item from its appearance and odour. They perceive that foods of acceptable organoleptic quality are also safe. They ignore the fact that many pathogens may exist, grow and produce toxins without changing the organoleptic quality of the food.

Among public health programmes, foodborne diseases have been perceived as mild and self-limiting. As a result, these diseases have received low priority in health programmes and no major efforts have been made to monitor their incidence and health consequences. Lack of information on the magnitude and consequences of these diseases has in turn resulted in a lack of appreciation of their real significance for health and the economy.

Too much or unbalanced information may also influence the public's perception of risks. In this context, the media play an important role. Over-publicizing the potential health effects of low-risk hazards may influence the risk perception of consumers and distract them from the high-risk ones. As policy-makers are obliged to respond to the concern of consumers, the risk perception of consumers may indirectly influence food safety programmes and government policy.

Failure to communicate scientifically identified risks and to offer options for controlling them allows ignorance, taboos and traditional belief to dictate people's behaviour and practices. Box 7 describes the elements of risk communication within the context of health education in food safety.

Box 7. Risk communication as related to health education in food safety

Food safety management has progressed rapidly in recent years. The current recommended approach involves risk analysis which includes risk assessment, risk management and risk communication (*27*).

Risk assessment is the scientific evaluation of known or potential adverse health effects resulting from human exposure to foodborne hazards. It involves identification and characterization of a hazard, and assessment of how likely it is that a health effect will result.

Risk management is the process of weighing policy alternatives for accepting, minimizing or reducing risks, and selecting and implementing appropriate options.

Risk communication is the exchange of information and opinions concerning risk and risk-related factors among risk assessors, risk managers and other interested parties.

The perception of what constitutes a risk depends on a person's culture, education and past experience. But while what is perceived as risk may differ, the basic scientific principles for dealing with risk are the same.

Risk communication, as a component of health education in food safety, consists of understanding consumers' perceptions of food safety risks and disseminating the results of risk assessment and decisions regarding risk management. The latter may include measures that governments or industries have to implement or practices that the public as consumers or food handlers should observe.

Effectiveness of education

There is no vaccine capable of providing general protection against foodborne diseases, and it is unlikely that there ever will be one. Vaccines are available only for hepatitis A, poliomyelitis and typhoid fever. As far as is economically possible, food service and catering establishments are encouraged to ensure the vaccination of their food handlers against hepatitis A (*39*). Attempts are being made to develop vaccines for other specific foodborne diseases such as shigellosis, rotavirus and enterotoxigenic *E. coli* (ETEC). However, these efforts are still at the research stage. Two oral cholera vaccines are also available in some countries, but they are recommended mainly for travellers. Present agricultural and animal husbandry practices cannot ensure that foodstuffs are free from contamination. Decontamination by processing is possible only for certain foods and certain pathogens and does not prevent recontamination during preparation. Also, many pathogens are transmitted to food by infected or colonized food handlers. To prevent the transmission of pathogens to foods by food handlers, the public health code in some countries requires persons to undergo a medical examination or some form of screening before they can be employed in food service establishments or as vendors of foods. Periodic testing of food workers is also frequently required. However, a cost–benefit analysis has shown that such measures are of limited value. WHO has recommended that resources should rather be used for the education and training of food handlers (*40*).

Food control authorities cannot intervene in every household. Also, inspection of food service establishments is not frequent enough to ensure consistent food safety. Therefore education and training in food safety remain the most important and effective options for the prevention of foodborne illnesses.

Experience from educational programmes on other health concerns, such as nutrition and dental hygiene, has shown that education, provided that it is well designed and implemented, is a feasible and cost-effective means of improving health status. Compared with other forms of intervention, health education is relatively cheap but produces long-lasting changes in the health-related behaviour of target groups (*41*).

Studies on the effectiveness of food safety education are scarce. Perhaps one of the most important examples is the reduction of listeriosis in several industrialized countries following the education of pregnant women. For example, in the USA industry and regulatory agencies took concerted measures, with a strong educational component for pregnant women, that were successful in reducing the number of cases of illness and deaths due to listeriosis by 44% and 48% respectively between 1989 and 1993 (*5*). Similar decreases as a result of the combined efforts of industry and government have been observed in the United Kingdom and some other countries (*6*).

The fall in the incidence of foodborne diseases observed in some Latin American countries after the outbreak of the cholera epidemic in the early 1990s, can also be attributed to a great extent to the intensive educational activities that took place as a result of the epidemic (see Fig. 3).

In Tunisia, as a result of intensive education of food handlers, the authorities succeeded in decreasing the incidence of diarrhoeal diseases among tourists from 40–54% in the 1980s to 27–37% in 1992 (*42, 43*).

An important example of the success of health education in food safety was the world fair "EXPO 92" in Seville, Spain, in 1992. Given the size of the event, the very complex organization of the fair, and the fact that it took place during the hot season in ambient temperatures up to 40 °C, the public health services faced a tremendous challenge. Education and training of food handlers in the food service establishments were, however, effective in preventing foodborne diseases. During the six months of EXPO 92, although tens of millions of meals were consumed, no significant report of foodborne illness was received (see Box 18, p. 107) (*44*).

Several studies have also demonstrated that the training and education of managers of food service establishments and food handlers lead to improved sanitary conditions in food service establishments and better scores during inspection (*45, 46*). Similarly, the training and education of food handlers in food safety assurance techniques following an outbreak of salmonellosis in an airline catering operation in Greece substantially improved the hygienic quality of the foods (see also page 51). In Jamaica, health education provided through the mass media was successful in preventing veno-occlusive disease of the liver caused by bush tea and ackee poisoning due to unripe ackee (*47*).

Conditions in developing countries

A polluted environment, lack of safe water supply and poor sanitation increase the likelihood of food contamination. Such conditions prevail in poor social settings, but they may also result from natural or man-made disasters (such as wars). Where the environment is polluted and food is likely to be con-taminated, it is all the more important to educate consumers and food handlers so that they can take specific measures to render food (including drinking-water) safe.

In countries where food control is weak because of lack of resources, education of consumers in food safety gives them the knowledge to be selective when choosing food and to refuse food that is of doubtful hygienic quality. A discriminating attitude by consumers can be effective in encouraging good manufacturing practices for commercially produced foods and can play an important role in improving food safety standards.

Foodborne diseases: preventable diseases

Most foodborne diseases are preventable. Measures for the control of most hazards are known. They are simple and can be applied by consumers or food handlers themselves. For many foodborne illnesses, health education in food safety is the most important option for prevention. While health education plays a very important role in preventing foodborne illnesses, it should be seen as part of a wider health promotion approach. This requires the participation of many sectors involved in the food chain and the development of healthy public policies, supportive environments and informed communities. It is regrettable, and even irresponsible, on the part of those who are in a position to change or influence the situation, if lives are endangered because adequate measures to inform and educate consumers or train food handlers have not been taken.

References

1. Jacob M. Salmonella in poultry: is there a solution? *Environmental policy and practice*, 1995, 5(2):75–80.

2. Roberts D. Sources of infection: food. *Lancet*, 1990, 336:859–861.

3. Tylleskär TM et al. Cassava cyanogens and konzo, an upper motoneurone disease found in Africa. *Lancet*, 1992, 339:208–211.

4. *The role of food safety in health and development. Report of a Joint FAO/WHO Expert Committee on Food Safety*. Geneva, World Health Organization, 1984 (WHO Technical Report Series, No. 705).

5. Tappero JW et al. Reduction in the incidence of human listeriosis in the United States: effectiveness of prevention efforts? *Journal of the American Medical Association*, 1995, 273(14):1118–1122.

6. McLauchlin J. The role of the Public Health Laboratory Service in England and Wales in the investigation of human listeriosis during the 1980s and 1990s. *Food control*, 1996, 7(4/5):235–239.

7. Esrey SA. Interventions for the control of diarrhoeal diseases among young children: improving water supplies and excreta disposal facilities. *Bulletin of the World Health Organization*, 1985, 63(4):757–772.

8. Bern C et al. The magnitude of the global problem of diarrhoeal disease: a ten year update. *Bulletin of the World Health Organization*, 1992, 70(6):705–714.

9. Guilford CT. *Integration of consumer interest in food control in developing countries. FAO Expert Consultation on Integration of Consumer Interests in Food Control, Rome, 14–18 June 1993*. Rome, Food and Agriculture Organization of the United Nations, 1993.

10. Gerba CP et al. Sensitive populations: who is at the greatest risk? *International journal of food microbiology*, 1996, 30:113–123.

11. Levine WC et al. Foodborne disease outbreaks in nursing homes, 1975 through 1987. *Journal of the American Medical Association*, 1991, 266(15):2105–2109.

12. Hlady WG, Mullen RC, Hopkin RS. *Vibrio vulnificus* from raw oysters. Leading cause of reported deaths from foodborne illness in Florida. *Journal of the Florida Medical Association*, 1993, 80(8):536–538.

13. Kotloff KL et al. Diarrhoeal morbidity during the first two years of life among HIV infected infants. *Journal of the American Medical Association*, 1994, 271(6):448–452.

14. Pavia AT et al. Diarrhoea among African children born to human immunodeficiency virus 1-infected mothers: clinical, microbiologic and epidemiologic features. *Pediatric infectious disease journal*, 1992, 11(12):996–1003.

15. *Food allergy and other adverse reactions to food*. Brussels, International Life Sciences Institute Europe, 1994.

16. Anderson JA. Allergic reactions to foods. *Critical reviews in food science and nutrition*, 1996, 36(S):S19–S38.

17. *Biotechnology and food safety. Report of a joint FAO/WHO consultation.* Rome, Food and Agriculture Organization of the United Nations, 1996 (Food and Agriculture Nutrition Paper 61).

18. *Report of the FAO Technical Consultation on Food Allergies.* Rome, Food and Agriculture Organization of the United Nations, 1995.

19. Ford GR, Horrocks CL. Hazard of microwave cooking: direct thermal damage to the pharynx and larynx. *Journal of laryngology and otology,* 1994, 108(6):509–510.

20. Budd R. Burns associated with the use of microwave ovens. *Journal of microwave power and electromagnetic energy,* 1992, 27(3):160–163.

21. Shukla PC. Ocular burn from microwaved egg. *Pediatric emergency care,* 1994, 10(4):229–231.

22. Lunden A, Uggla A. Infectivity of *Toxoplasma gondii* in mutton following curing, smoking, freezing or microwave cooking. *International journal of food microbiology,* 1992, 15:357–363.

23. Coote PJ, Holyoak CD, Cole MB. Thermal inactivation of *Listeria monocytogenes* during a process of simulating temperatures achieved during microwave heating. *Journal of applied bacteriology,* 1991, 70(6):489–494.

24. Bates CJ, Spencer RC. Survival of *Salmonella* species in eggs poached using a microwave oven. *Journal of hospital infection,* 1995, 29(2):121–127.

25. Heddleson RA, Doores S. Injury of *Salmonella* species heated by microwave energy. *Journal of food protection,* 1994, 57(12):1068–1073.

26. Gessner BD, Beller M. Protective effect of conventional cooking versus use of microwave ovens in an outbreak of salmonellosis. *American journal of epidemiology,* 1994, 139(9):903–909.

27. Evans MR, Parry SM, Ribeiro CD. *Salmonella* outbreak from microwave cooked food. *Epidemiology and infection,* 1995, 115(2):227–230.

28. Blundell JE et al. *Light foods.* Brussels, International Life Sciences Institute Europe, 1995.

29. Lee K. Food neophobia: major causes and treatments. *Food technology,* 1989, December, 62–73.

30. Oltersdorf U. Differences in German consumer concerns over suggested health and food hazards. In: Feichtinger E, Köhler BM, eds. *Current research into eating practices. Contribution of social sciences. 16th Annual Scientific Meeting of AGEV, Postdam, Germany, 14–16 October 1993.* Supplement to *Ernährungs-Umschau (Nutrition Survey),* 1995, 42:171–173.

31. *Application of risk analysis to food standards issues. Report of the Joint FAO/WHO Expert Consultation, Geneva, Switzerland, 13–17 March 1995.* Geneva, World Health Organization, 1995 (unpublished document WHO/FNU/FOS/95.3; available on request from Food Safety, World Health Organization, 1211 Geneva 27, Switzerland).

32. Weiss MG. Cultural models of diarrhoeal illness: conceptual framework and review. *Social science and medicine,* 1988, 27:5–16.

33. Bukenya GB et al. The relationship of mothers' perception of babies' faeces and other factors to childhood diarrhoea in an urban settlement of Papua New Guinea. *Annals of tropical paediatrics*, 1990, 10:185–189.

34. Ahmed IS et al. Knowledge, attitudes and practices of mothers regarding diarrhoea among children in a Sudanese rural community. *East African medical journal*, 1994, 71(11):716–719.

35. Mortimore SE. *How effective are the current sources of food hygiene and education and training in shaping behaviour?* [Thesis]. Leicester, University of Leicester Centre for Labour Market Studies, 1993.

36. Pelto GH. The role of behavioral research in the prevention and management of invasive diarrhoeas. *Reviews of infectious diseases*, 1991, 13(Suppl. 4):S255–S258.

37. Zeitlyn S, Islam F. The use of soap and water in two Bangladeshi communities: implications for transmission of diarrhoea. *Reviews of infectious diseases*, 1991, 13(Suppl. 4):S259–S264.

38. Weinstein ND. Unrealistic optimism about susceptibility to health problems. *Journal of behaviour medicine*, 1982, 5(4):441–460.

39. Prevention of foodborne hepatitis A. *Weekly epidemiological record*, 1993, 68(5):25–26.

40. *Health surveillance and management procedures for food-handling personnel. Report of a WHO Consultation.* Geneva, World Health Organization, 1989 (WHO Technical Report Series, No. 785).

41. Ashworth A, Feachem RG. Interventions for the control of diarrhoeal diseases among young children: weaning education. *Bulletin of the World Health Organization*, 1985, 63:1115–1127.

42. Steffen R. *Anfallsrate der Reisediarrhoe bei Schweizer Touristen in Tunesien, 1992. [Rates of travellers' diarrhoea among Swiss tourists in Tunisia, 1992.]* [Thesis]. Zurich, University of Zurich. 1994.

43. Cartwright RY, Chahed M. Foodborne diseases in travellers. *World health statistics quarterly*, 50(1/2):102–110.

44. Duran-Moreno A, Moreno-Duran A, Toledano-Hidalgo P. El control de la higiene alimentaria durante la Exposicion Universal de Sevilla (EXPO '92). [Control of food hygiene during the world's fair in Seville, EXPO '92.] *Gaceta sanitaria*, 1993, 7(38):249–258.

45. Penninger HK, Rodman VA. Food service managerial certification: how effective has it been? *Dairy and food sanitation*, 1984, 4(7):260–264.

46. Mathias RG et al. The effects of inspection frequency and food handler education on restaurant inspection violations. *Canadian journal of public health*, 1995, 86(1):46–50.

47. *Health education in food safety. Report of a WHO consultation* (unpublished document WHO/EHE/FOS/88.7; available on request from Food Safety, World Health Organization, 1211 Geneva 27, Switzerland).

CHAPTER 3

Approaches for selection of key behaviours

It is often necessary to focus an educational programme on a selected number of positive behaviours. These are chosen because changing them is likely to have a significant positive impact on health or because they have the potential to prevent a specific foodborne disease cost-effectively. Such behaviours are referred to here as "key behaviours".

The selection of key behaviours—i.e. behaviours which need to be changed or reinforced—is one of the most fundamental concerns in any health education programme. In food safety, selection of key behaviours is more complex than in other areas of health education such as the prevention of smoking where the educational programme addresses one hazard (e.g. nicotine) and basically one type of behaviour (e.g. refraining from smoking). The difficulty in the selection of key behaviours in food safety stems from several factors.

- Education in food safety is often aimed at preventing a wide range of diseases with various etiological agents: bacteria, viruses, parasites, naturally occurring toxins, and other hazardous chemical agents and antinutritional factors.

- The etiological agents differ in behaviour and ecology. Some, like most bacteria, grow on food, while others such as viruses and parasites do not. Bacteria alone show a wealth of variation. The range of temperature for bacterial growth varies widely. Some agents, such as salmonellae, are mesophyllic and their growth is slowed down or stopped at refrigeration temperatures (below 10 °C); others such as *Listeria monocytogenes* or *Yersinia enterocolitica* can grow at these temperatures. While bacteria survive freezing, most parasites are killed by thorough freezing (−18 °C for at least 24 hours). Some agents, like *Vibrio cholerae*, are sensitive to acids and may not survive an acidic food environment or even gastric acid, while others such as *E. coli* O157:H7 are acid-resistant. Some bacteria grow or produce toxin only under anaerobic conditions, while others require oxygen. Some bacteria are hazardous if ingested (e.g. *Campylobacter*), while others are hazardous only if they have had the opportunity to produce toxin in food (e.g. *Clostridium botulinum*[1]). The toxin of some bacteria (e.g. *Clostridium botulinum*) is thermolabile and is destroyed by adequate heating, whereas the toxin of some

---

[1] For infants under the age of one year, the ingestion of *Clostridium botulinum* cells may be dangerous as it may lead to infant botulism.

others (e.g. *Staphylococcus aureus*) is heat-resistant. There may be variation even within one species. For example, *Bacillus cereus* may produce heat-labile or heat-stable toxins.

● Food preparation is a complex procedure that involves a multitude of actions, some influenced by socioeconomic conditions or cultural habits. Not only may the actions themselves be hazardous (e.g. undercooking, storing at room temperature, touching food with contaminated hands) but the order in which they are carried out may constitute a risk factor. For example, in cases of diarrhoeal disease in Kiambu, a district on the outskirts of Nairobi, Kenya, it was found that the cause of food contamination was the addition of raw milk or leftovers from earlier meals after the final cooking process. This reintroduced pathogens into the food. The same action prior to cooking may have not been hazardous (*1*).

● The likelihood of contamination, and thus the risk that a certain food or behaviour will causes disease, varies according to environmental conditions (including pollution and climate change) and source of food. For example, the consumption of raw vegetables that have been fertilized with untreated manure or wastewater may present a health hazard, but if vegetables are grown according to good agricultural practice they are generally safe. In times of algal bloom, or "red tide" in the sea, the consumption of shellfish or some species of fish may present a greater health risk than in normal circumstances. Thus, a type of food or method of preparation may be safe at one time, or in one area, but unsafe at other times or in other environmental conditions.

● The infective dose or toxic level varies according to pathogens, toxic substances, individuals and the food matrix. Some pathogens, such as *Shigella* spp., have a low infective dose, and even a few cells can cause disease. Others, such as *V. cholerae* or *Salmonellae* (non-*typhi*), may require a large number of cells to cause infection, and healthy adults are at risk only if the food is grossly contaminated or has been subject to time–temperature abuse. Even pathogens with a generally high infective dose may sometimes present a danger to health in low numbers if the composition or structure of the food is likely to protect them from gastric acid. For example, ingestion of less than 50 cells of *S. napoli* in a chocolate bar caused an outbreak of salmonellosis in the United Kingdom because of the protective effects of the lipid component (*2*). In a nationwide outbreak of salmonellosis in Germany, caused by contaminated paprika and paprika powder, it was shown that even relatively low numbers of salmonellae adapted to dry conditions could cause illness (*3*). The risk posed by foodborne diseases is not the same for all individuals. Certain individuals are more vulnerable to some pathogens than other individuals. Thus, a food or behaviour may constitute a risk factor for one person but not for another. In addition, some persons may have allergies to some foods or ingredients, while others are not affected.

These factors are often interrelated and are also influenced by socioeconomic conditions and culture. This interrelation is illustrated by an example of an outbreak of cholera in an African village. During an epidemic of cholera in Mali in 1984, during which 1793 people were affected and 406 persons died, the epidemiological investigations identified leftover millet gruel as one of the routes of transmission. This gruel, a staple of the Sahel diet, was usually prepared once a day and commonly eaten without reheating. The gruel was usually acidified by the addition of curdled goat's milk, which made the survival and growth of *V. cholerae* unlikely. However, it is believed that during that epidemic this milk was in scant supply because of drought. In the absence of curdled goat's milk, the millet gruel supported the growth of *V. cholerae* at ambient temperature (*4*). This shows how a change in the macro-environment (drought), hand-in-hand with socioeconomic factors (lack of refrigeration to keep food cold, lack of fuel to keep it hot or reheat it, and a polluted environment leading to the presence of *V. cholerae* in food), influenced the micro-environment of the pathogen (acidity) and led to the survival and growth of *V. cholerae*. Thus a common behaviour (keeping and eating leftover food without further heat treatment) which was traditionally safe became hazardous.

There is a need to reflect on the kinds of behaviour on which food handlers and consumers need to be trained and educated. It is difficult to change behavioural patterns and it should be attempted only if a positive and clear health effect can be expected.

Below are some of the approaches that have been used for identifying risk factors for foodborne disease and key behaviours which should be the subject of health education. Each approach has merits and limitations. Some suit certain situations better than others. Sometimes a combination of approaches may be used. The approaches described below mainly identify practices that are important from the point of view of food safety. They do not necessarily determine the cultural, socioeconomic and personal factors that lead to the behaviour in question. To understand what motivates people to adopt a certain behaviour it is important to combine the technical information collected through these approaches with data from anthropological and behavioural studies that investigate people's knowledge, practice and constraints (*5*). These latter types of studies are briefly described on pages 82–84. For more in-depth information, readers are recommended to refer to other literature dealing with this area (*6, 7*).

Selection of behaviour

Toxicological or epidemiological evidence of hazards inherent in certain foods

Toxicological or epidemiological studies provide evidence of the potential hazards associated with certain foods, such as toxicants in mushrooms or wild green plants, marine biotoxins in fishery products, and haemagglutinin (lectins) in red kidney beans.

In areas where foods known to be potentially hazardous constitute an important part of the diet, the population should be informed and educated on how to protect themselves (Box 8). Where the hazards in foodstuffs cannot be eliminated by suitable preparation, people should be educated to recognize and avoid them. In other cases, people should be advised to apply the necessary and appropriate practices during preparation in order to eliminate the hazard. Educational intervention could be intensified at times when the risk of exposure of the population to a potentially toxic food increases. For instance, climatic conditions may lead to an increase in the number of toxic food mushrooms, or toxic algae.

Change in dietary habits may also be related to increased exposure. For instance, in Denmark, the influence of immigrants led to an increase in the consumption of red kidney beans among the local population.

Box 8. Behaviour promoted for prevention of mushroom poisoning in Denmark (9)

Five hints about mushrooms
For people who want to pick and eat wild mushrooms

■ Eat mushrooms that you are 100% sure of.

■ Eat only recognized edible mushrooms.

■ Use only fresh mushrooms for cooking; refrigerate leftovers immediately.

■ Always start with a small portion of a new, edible mushroom. Possible hypersensitivity will then be a less painful event.

■ Don't eat wild mushrooms raw, as many wild mushrooms may lead to unpleasant reactions when eaten raw.

As the indigenous population was not familiar with the proper preparation of the beans, the number of cases of intoxication due to haemagglutinin increased. Subsequently, the health authorities in Denmark launched a campaign to educate consumers in the proper cooking of various beans. Posters giving information on the cooking times needed to inhibit lectins in beans were produced and distributed to consumers. Similar initiatives were also taken to prevent mushroom intoxication (Box 8) and illness due to solanine in green potatoes (*8–11*).

Monitoring contaminants

Monitoring of contaminants is a prospective approach, in which information on the extent and level of hazardous contaminants and their potential health risk is obtained by monitoring foodstuffs for contaminants. This information then provides the basis for regulatory action or for informing and educating the public. Such an approach is particularly important for chemical contaminants (e.g. toxic metals) that may enter the food chain through the environment. In Sweden, monitoring of methylmercury in lake fish indicated high levels of this toxic metal. As a result of the monitoring programme, the population, particularly pregnant women, was advised to limit consumption of some species of fish (e.g. perch, pike, turbot, eel, halibut) in order to keep dietary intake of methylmercury within safe limits.

When disasters such as nuclear accidents occur, the monitoring of contaminants is of the utmost importance so that the population can be advised which foods may have been contaminated and which should be avoided. This approach is also often used in programmes for the prevention of paralytic shellfish poisoning (PSP) and other seafood poisoning. Several countries carry out monitoring programmes for PSP, and when the level of toxins in the edible portion of the shellfish exceeds safe levels, the area in which the shellfish grow is closed and the public is advised accordingly (*12*). Countries such as Canada also carry out a toxic phytoplankton monitoring programme to prevent domoic acid poisoning.

The results of monitoring have also been useful in the education of consumers on the problem of using glazed tableware which leaches toxic metals. Some ceramic products are coated with a glaze that may contain toxic metals such as lead or cadmium. These metals can leach from the glaze into food, particularly acidic food (*13*). Many countries have no legislative controls regarding leachable metals in glazed tableware.

In Mexico, use of lead-glazed ceramics for storage of drinks or cooking has been reported to cause high levels of lead in blood in some persons (*14–17*). In Australia, imported tableware products are routinely monitored by the customs service, and consumers are educated about the dangers associated with using "souvenir" or antique pottery for food (*18*). In Geneva, Switzerland, monitoring of tableware for lead has shown that 23% in 1992 and 10% in 1995 contained levels of lead above authorized limits. To protect consumers, food

---

Box 9. Mystery poisonings traced to lead in cups (*19*)

Donald Wallace and his wife Frances each drank 8–10 cups of coffee a day from poorly made terracotta cups they had purchased while on holiday. They were both consuming lead that was leaching in excessive amounts from the cups and over a three-year period they became sick. Their doctors were unable to diagnose their illness correctly at first.

---

control authorities provide a service to which consumers can bring their table-ware for testing (see also Box 9).

Monitoring ready-to-eat foods from food service establishments or street vendors for biological contaminants provides information on safe handling. While such information by itself does not provide an indication of inappropriate behaviour, it indicates the services that need to be further investigated and receive advice. The population may be advised to avoid places where food is likely to be unsafe. Monitoring the safety of street-vended foods in areas surrounding schools or hospitals may be important in certain countries, since outbreaks of foodborne disease have repeatedly occurred in schoolchildren consuming food from street vendors.

Epidemiological investigation and review of foodborne disease outbreaks

Outbreaks are opportunities to learn about the epidemiology of diseases and their risk factors. Thus, epidemiological investigation of foodborne disease outbreaks can be used to identify errors in food handling (Box 10).

The merit of this approach is that it allows the main factors leading to foodborne diseases in a population to be identified and ranked according to their importance by disease, type of food implicated, and location where food is contaminated or consumed. For example, reviews of foodborne disease outbreaks in several countries have shown that the major risk factor for salmonellosis is time–temperature abuse, while for shigellosis and typhoid fever it is the handling of food by an infected food handler (*20*).

This approach is also instrumental in identifying places (e.g. food service or catering establishments) where foodborne disease outbreaks are likely to occur. Managers and employees of such establishments should be the targets of education interventions.

Box 10. Investigating foodborne disease outbreaks (*20, 21*)

Investigation of foodborne disease outbreaks in both industrialized and developing countries has indicated errors in food handling that are leading factors in the cause of foodborne disease. Factors that are predominant causes of foodborne disease outbreaks and that should be the subject of health education measures are:

− preparation of food several hours before consumption, combined with storage at temperatures that favour the growth of pathogenic bacteria and/or formation of toxins;

− insufficient cooking or reheating of food to reduce or eliminate pathogens;

− use of contaminated water or raw food material;

− cross-contamination in the premises where food is prepared;

− infected or colonized persons in charge of the preparation of meals.

The limitation of this approach is that in most countries, particularly developing countries, the infrastructure and trained personnel for investigation of foodborne disease outbreaks are poor or non-existent. Also, usually only outbreaks involving large numbers of people are investigated. Thus, statistics may not adequately reflect incorrect food handling leading to foodborne disease outbreaks in households. Rarely, if at all, are cases of infant diarrhoea in households investigated.

Case–control studies of sporadic cases

Case–control epidemiological studies of sporadic cases are widely used to study risk factors and thus identify behaviours that need to be changed or promoted (*22*). Case–control studies can be relatively simple and economical to carry out. However, the validity of the factors identified and the success in targeting the relevant risk factors depend very much on how the study is designed. As studies become more comprehensive, the validity of the results improves but the expense and the complexity increase considerably. In a case–control study, a group of people with a particular disease are interviewed about their behaviour and practices, and the results are compared with those from interviews with a suitable control group of people not affected by the disease. Such studies have been used, for example, to investigate the risk factors for foodborne toxoplasmosis (*23*) and diarrhoeal diseases (*24–31*).

Unfortunately, many studies omit factors related to food safety or do not reflect them properly. As a result, conclusions may be misleading.

The Hazard Analysis and Critical Control Point system

The Hazard Analysis and Critical Control Point (HACCP) system is a rational and scientific method of food safety assurance. It consists of systematic identification and assessment of hazards and determination of effective control measures. A full HACCP system is based on seven principles (Box 11).

Although the seventh principle (documentation and record-keeping) is essential for food processing operations, it is not applicable in homes and it may not be feasible in street vending operations. In certain types of food service establishments, full documentation and record-keeping may also be limited. The application of the sixth principle may also present some difficulties. However, the first five principles are crucial in health education. The HACCP system was originally developed to ensure the safety of foods for astronauts. It was later adopted by food industries as a method of safety assurance for ensuring the safety of processed and manufactured food. Today the HACCP system is applied across the entire food chain from primary production, processing and manufacturing to final preparation and consumption of foods—including foods

---

Box 11. The HACCP system: principles and definitions (*32*)

1. Conduct hazard analysis (i.e. identify hazard, evaluate risk and specify measures for risk control).

   Hazard: A biological, chemical or physical agent or factor with the potential to cause an adverse health effect.

2. Determine critical control points (CCPs).

   Critical control point: A step at which control can be applied that is essential to prevent or eliminate a food safety hazard or reduce it to an acceptable level.

3. Establish critical limits at each CCP.

   Critical limit: A criterion which separates acceptability from unacceptability.

4. Establish monitoring procedures.

   Monitoring: The act of conducting a planned sequence of observations or measurements of control of parameters to assess whether a CCP is under control.

5. Establish corrective actions.

   Corrective action: Actions to be taken when the results of monitoring the CCP indicate a loss of control.

6. Establish verification procedures.

   Verification: The application of methods, procedures or tests, in addition to those used in monitoring, to determine compliance with the HACCP plan and/or whether the HACCP plan needs modification.

7. Establish documentation procedures.

---

prepared in households and in food service and catering establishments, as well as street foods. In the context of this book, the HACCP system has two major applications. The system is both a method of safety assurance in the preparation of foods in food service and catering establishments, and a tool for the selection of key behaviours that can be the focus of educational interventions.

With adequate training in the HACCP system, managers and food handlers will be able to assess the food preparation process critically, identify the hazards associated with each step, and adopt measures (and if necessary modify the process) to ensure the safety of the food being prepared. The HACCP system enables managers of food service establishments and food handlers to judge what needs to be done in each situation and to decide whether:

— all measures necessary for ensuring food safety have been taken into consideration;
— all measures are implemented at the appropriate step in the food preparation process;
— all measures are implemented correctly.

Similarly, the HACCP approach can be used by food inspectors to carry out a more efficient inspection of food premises, concentrating their attention and resources on the most critical parts of the food preparation process (Box 12).

The application of the HACCP system to foods prepared in mass catering establishments has, in many instances, proven to be efficient in improving hygiene and preventing foodborne diseases. Adoption of the HACCP system by an airline catering establishment in Greece, following an outbreak of salmonellosis in 1991, substantially improved the hygienic quality of the food (*33*).

Foods prepared in homes, street food vending operations and food service catering establishments may be studied with an HACCP-based approach (*34–37*). This will lead to identification of practices that are necessary to control hazards in the food (i.e. control measures) at each step in food preparation, and also identification of the steps in the food preparation where control is essential to ensure safety (critical control points). The control measures at the critical control points should be the focus of educational programmes. Food handlers should be trained to implement these measures correctly and should also learn what to do with the food if the conditions have not been met.

Fig. 11 shows a flow diagram for

Box 12. Food inspection and the HACCP system

The HACCP system has major benefits for food inspectors who control food service and catering establishments. The HACCP system overcomes the limitations of traditional approaches to food control, such as:

– the difficulty in collecting and examining sufficient samples to obtain meaningful representative information;

– the length of time required to obtain the results (in many cases, by the time the results are obtained the consumer may have already eaten the food);

– the high cost of end-product testing and recalling products if there is evidence of contamination;

– insufficient accuracy of inspection techniques in predicting food safety problems that may arise as a result of change in recipe and/or food preparation procedure.

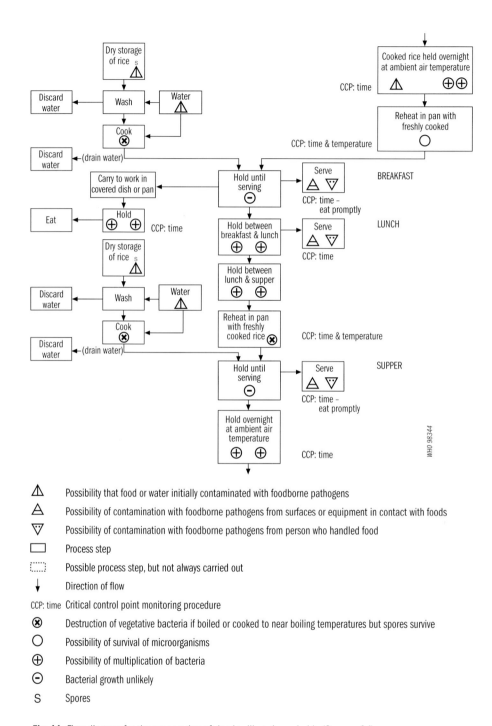

⚠	Possibility that food or water initially contaminated with foodborne pathogens
△	Possibility of contamination with foodborne pathogens from surfaces or equipment in contact with foods
▽	Possibility of contamination with foodborne pathogens from person who handled food
▭	Process step
⬚	Possible process step, but not always carried out
↓	Direction of flow
CCP: time	Critical control point monitoring procedure
⊗	Destruction of vegetative bacteria if boiled or cooked to near boiling temperatures but spores survive
○	Possibility of survival of microorganisms
⊕	Possibility of multiplication of bacteria
⊖	Bacterial growth unlikely
S	Spores

Fig. 11. Flow diagram for the preparation of rice in village households (Source: *34*)

the preparation of rice in a village household. The application of the HACCP system to the preparation of rice showed that storage of cooked rice was a critical control point in the preparation of rice, and that households should learn to store the food safely by observing the time–temperature conditions of storage. Households should be taught to keep the cooked rice cold (below 10 °C), or hot (near or above 60 °C), or eat it without delay. If these conditions are not met, the rice should be discarded. Thorough reheating may also reduce the risk of intoxication, although it does not provide total protection as some emetic toxins of *Bacillus cereus* are not affected by heat.

It is noteworthy that the results of such studies are usually consistent with the risk factors identified through epidemiological surveillance of foodborne diseases. Therefore, in countries where there is no functional epidemiological surveillance system, the HACCP approach presents a cost-effective alternative. Since the HACCP approach is based on observations of practices and analysis of hazards associated with every stage of an operation, the approach is likely to highlight food preparation habits that are specific to a certain culture or ethnic group and that are of significance for food safety. It enables behaviours to be identified in the socioeconomic and environmental context in which they occur. Thus, factors such as lack of safe water or sanitation, the presence of pets and household animals, and the health status of the consumer, all of which have bearings on food safety, will also be considered in the hazard analysis (principle 1). Hence, the HACCP approach is a particularly useful tool both for identifying risk factors for diarrhoeal diseases in developing countries and for identifying preventive measures.

WHO has pioneered the application of the HACCP system in cottage industries, food service establishments, street food vending operations and homes (*38*). Studies that have used the HACCP system to identify behaviour that should be targeted by health education have been carried out in several countries (e.g. Dominican Republic, Malaysia, Myanmar, Pakistan, Peru and Zambia) (*39–43*).

Factors underlying food-related behaviour

Behaviour is influenced by a number of cultural, socioeconomic and environmental factors, as well as by personal characteristics (e.g. knowledge). In social science these factors are classified as follows (*6, 44*):

● Predisposing factors are those antecedents to behaviour that provide the rationale or motivation for the behaviour (e.g. knowledge, beliefs, values, attitudes, confidence, existing skills).

● Enabling factors are the conditions in the environment which enable the motivation to be realized. Enabling factors may be availability, accessibility to facilities for food preparation (e.g. water for washing, fuel for cooking), or legal infrastructure such as maternal leave from the workplace which enables mothers to breastfeed and care for small children.

● Reinforcing factors are factors that follow a behaviour. They provide the continuing reward or incentive for the behaviour and contribute to its persistence or repetition (e.g. the attitude of managers of food service establishments towards food handlers who are vigilant in handling food safely, or the attitudes of food inspectors, family, peers or consumers). An example is rewarding a food service establishment (e.g. by awarding stars) on the basis of observed food hygiene, or by giving an award to food handlers who successfully pass an examination or test on food hygiene. It is certainly not reinforcement if a supervisor reprimands a food handler for spending time or resources on ensuring safety (e.g. washing).

In any health education programme, it is important to consider the influence of these three types of factor.

There are different methods for assessing cultural, socioeconomic and personal factors. These include "knowledge, attitude, practice" (KAP) studies, surveys, group discussions, interviews with key informants, participatory methods and so on. The use of some of these methods in relation to food safety is discussed briefly below.

Knowledge, attitude and practice studies

KAP studies have been used by some scientists to identify incorrect knowledge as well as beliefs, attitudes and practices which militate against food safety (Box 12).

The information collected through such studies is based on replies to a well-defined questionnaire. While KAP studies can give useful information about people's knowledge, beliefs and attitudes regarding specific aspects of food safety, their use in studying behaviour and practices may be limited because people do not always practice what they know, say or believe they should be doing. Therefore, the information collected through questionnaire-based surveys is of interest mainly for evaluating people's know-how and perception of foodborne hazards and risks. For studying patterns of food preparation and identifying practices which need to be implemented to ensure safety, the recommended approach is to use observational studies (although these may result in bias as people's behaviour may be different from normal if they are watched).

Relatively few KAP studies have been carried out in the area of food safety. However, one example is a KAP study that was conducted among persons working at a temporary public eating place at a three-day fair in the USA. The study focused on four factors that frequently contribute to outbreaks of foodborne illnesses—heat treatment (temperature control), time–temperature abuse dur-

---

Box 12. How knowledge, beliefs, values and attitude may affect food safety (Adapted from *6* and *44*)

Knowledge and skills

Knowledge is necessary before a conscious action can take place. However, the desired action may probably not occur until a person receives a hint strong enough to trigger the motivation to act on that knowledge. Knowledge can be gained through information provided by health professionals, parents, teachers, books, the mass media and other sources. It may also be gained through experience. At times it may also be necessary to verify the correctness of the knowledge of the population. For instance, people may not know that eggs are contaminated with salmonella, or that food is a potential source of agents that cause diarrhoeal disease. Skills may also predispose a person to act in a particular way. For instance, a mother who already possesses the skill to breastfeed is more likely to breastfeed her next child.

Beliefs

Belief is a conviction that a phenomenon or object is true or real. Beliefs are usually derived from parents, grandparents and other respected people. Beliefs are usually accepted without proof that they are true. For instance, in regard to breast milk, some people believe (wrongly) that colostrum should not be fed to babies. Some people also believe that contamination can be detected from the smell or appearance of food.

Values

Values tend to cluster within ethnic groups and across generations of people who share a common history and geographical identity. For instance, communities value the capacity of mothers to provide adequate nutritious and safe food for newborn children through breast milk.

Attitude

Attitudes reflect likes or dislikes towards certain categories of objects, persons, or situations. They often stem from our experiences or from those of people close to us. They attract us to things or make us wary of them. Attitudes are sometimes based on limited experience. Therefore people may form attitudes without understanding the whole situation. Communities may not wish to alter the preparation of traditional foods even when they are shown to be unsafe. Some food handlers may dislike being taught how to prepare food hygienically.

---

ing food storage, cross-contamination, and neglect of personal hygiene. The assessment of the workers revealed deficiencies in knowledge, attitude and practices with regard to the first three factors mentioned, despite the fact that some had been working for years at the fair and in other food service establishments. Also, even though the workers indicated hand-washing to be important in connection with food handling, only one person was observed washing his hands. Again, while all the workers knew that they should not touch cooked foods with their hands, 44% were observed doing so. In another study, 219 managers and owners of retail food markets were surveyed for their knowledge, opinions and practices regarding food safety. The results confirmed a distinct lack of fundamental knowledge about food handling (*45*). The results of another investigation of the impact of personnel knowledge on food safety practices in convenience stores also showed a clear correlation between the food safety standards maintained and the manager's knowledge of food safety (*46*).

A study of personal hygiene and food safety practices revealed serious deficiencies among Nigerian professional food handlers working in catering establishments for low-income groups. The lack of knowledge in a predominantly female workforce suggested equally low standards of domestic food hygiene. The study indicated that nearly half of food handlers did not wash their hands adequately before preparing food, about two-thirds did not report to the doctor when suffering from diarrhoea, and even fewer stopped working while suffering from diarrhoea or other symptoms of illness. In about 20% of cases, leftover food was kept at ambient temperature and in 50% of cases it was given to children and other relatives (*47*). KAP studies have also revealed discrepancies between what government officials think people know (or should know) and what in reality people do know and practice. A survey of people fishing on the catchment basins of Jamaica Bay Wildlife Refuge in New York City, USA, showed that of the 154 groups interviewed only 19% were convinced that the waters were contaminated and that fish were unsafe, despite state warnings to the contrary, and fisherman made nearly five visits per month and ate on average three fish a week. The remaining fish were eaten by their families. Most people believed that fish were safe to eat or that they could recognize if one was spoiled (*48*).

Surveys

Food safety surveys have been carried out by telephone or by observation. A telephone and observational survey in the USA, covering 7000 and 2130 people respectively, revealed disparities between the hand-washing behaviour of men and women. Across all cities where the survey was conducted, women washed their hands more often than men (74% versus 61%). The survey was part of a campaign that was designed to provide consumers with easy-to-understand information about the importance of hand-washing. Another telephone survey in the USA showed that, although 80% of the people interviewed knew the importance of preventing cross-contamination, only 67% washed or changed cutting boards after cutting up raw meat or poultry (*49*). Box 13 indicates similar findings in another study in the USA.

Surveys of knowledge and attitudes alone have been useful in assessing public knowledge or perceptions of new food technologies, emerging pathogens and risky foods, as well as of factors that underlie certain beliefs, attitudes and practices. For instance, a study in Denmark provided insight into consumers' worries about food safety and the basis for their food choices. It revealed that few consumers felt that they had accurate knowledge of food safety issues (*51*). A study in Germany indicated an obvious lack of concern for and knowledge of the rules of proper hygiene during daily household activities, particularly among single persons and younger segments of the population. The study showed that a great proportion of the German population does not properly control the temperature of the refrigerator, does not know the importance of proper stirring during reheating of food in microwave ovens, and is unaware of the need to separate perishable and other foods during storage. More importantly, too many people in the study believed they could identify contaminated foods by taste, smell or appearance (*52*).

In a study in New Zealand, awareness of key food safety practices was assessed in 244 persons. The study showed that only a few respondents were completely familiar with all the correct food safety practices and generally found difficulty in differentiating between examples of safe and unsafe food handling (*53*).

A major interview study was conducted in 1991 throughout the European Community. Respondents' knowledge about and attitudes towards a range of new technologies, including biotechnology, were investigated. The study demonstrated a positive correlation between optimism regarding the potential benefits of biotechnology and knowledge. It also revealed some demographic differences: males had more knowledge than females, and younger people tended to know more than older people. A survey was also conducted in the USA to determine consumer attitudes to food irradiation. Results indicated that 72% of consumers were aware of irradiation but over 30% believed that

Box 13. Results of a study carried out in the USA on the prevalence of risky food consumption or food preparation behaviour (*50*)

Behaviour	Positive reply %
Consuming raw foods of animal origin	
● raw eggs	53
● steak tartare	5
● undercooked hamburgers	23
● raw clams and oysters	17
● raw sushi or ceviche	8
Use of cutting board without cleaning after exposure to raw poultry or meat	26

irradiated food is radioactive. At least 45% of consumers stated that they would be irradiated by such food (*54*).

Other methods

One method that has been found to be useful in investigating people's attitudes, beliefs and perceptions is the focus group discussion. Focus groups are informal sessions in which representatives of the target population (8–12 persons) are asked to discuss their thoughts on a specific subject. Focus groups are valuable in investigating cultural, socioeconomic and personal information about a subject and can also be used in developing educational programmes (e.g. by testing an educational message) (*55*). In the USA, researchers used this method to help the Department of Agriculture to develop an effective label format for raw and partially cooked meat and poultry products. As a result of this exercise, the authorities made a number of revisions to the label format to take into account the understanding and preferences of the users (*56, 57*).

Participatory methods seek a community's participation in the collection of data. There are a number of approaches. One is the Participatory Hygiene and Sanitation Transformation (PHAST). This method has been used to improve hygienic behaviour related to water and sanitation in a number of countries, e.g. Botswana, Kenya, Uganda and Zimbabwe (*58*). The method uses drawings to focus people's discussions. Various "tools" and "activities" are structured for particular purposes, such as "three-pile sorting" of 15–30 drawings to analyse whether existing hygiene behaviours are good or bad. Some tools are designed to raise awareness, while others are for investigation, data collection and analysis. The methodology also has activities for planning actions and for the monitoring and evaluation of change. Participatory methods aim to raise self-esteem and to help people feel ownership of the decisions. The methods are particularly successful in getting women to participate in cultures where they would traditionally not participate, and in getting illiterate people involved.

References

1. Pertet AM et al. Weaning food hygiene in Kiambu, Kenya. In: Alnwick S et al., eds. *Improving young child feeding in eastern and southern Africa: household-level food technology. Proceedings of a workshop held in Nairobi, Kenya, 12–16 October 1987.* Ottawa, International Development Research Centre, 1988:234–239.

2. Greenwood MA, Hooper WL. Chocolate bars contaminated with *Salmonella napoli*: an infectivity study. *British medical journal*, 1983, 266:1394.

3. Lehmacher A, Bockemühl J, Aleksic S. Nationwide outbreak of human salmonellosis in Germany due to contaminated paprika and paprika-powdered potato chips. *Epidemiology and infection*, 1995, 115:501–511.

4. Tauxe VR et al. Epidemic cholera in Mali: high mortality and multiple routes of transmission in a famine area. *Epidemiology and infection*, 1988, 100:279–289.

5. *Report of the Task Force on Health Education.* Geneva, World Health Organization, 1990 (unpublished document WHO/HPP/FOS/90.3; available on request from Department of Health Promotion, World Health Organization, 1211 Geneva 27, Switzerland).

6. Green L, Kreuter MW. *Health promotion planning. An educational and environmental approach.* Mountain View, CA, Mayfield Publishing Company, 1991.

7. Almedom AM, Blumenthal U, Manderson L. *Hygiene evaluation procedures. Approaches and methods for assessing water- and sanitation-ralated hygiene practices.* Boston, MA, International Nutrition Foundation for Developing Countries, 1997.

8. *Bonner: skal tilberedes rigtigt-ellers kan de vaere skadelige. [Beans should be properly prepared, otherwise they can be harmful.]* Copenhagen, National Food Agency [poster].

9. *Ka de spises? [Can they be eaten?]* Copenhagen, National Food Agency [poster].

10. *En heldig kartoffel. [A lucky potato.]* Copenhagen, National Food Agency [poster].

11. *Health education in food safety. Report of a WHO consultation.* Geneva, World Health Organization, 1988 (unpublished document WHO/EHE/FOS/88.87; available on request from Food Safety, World Health Organization, 1211 Geneva 27, Switzerland).

12. *Aquatic marine and freshwater biotoxins.* Geneva, World Health Organization, 1984 (Environmental Health Criteria, No. 37).

13. *Safe use of lead glazes for foodware.* New York, International Lead Zinc Research Organization Inc., 1979.

14. Rojas-Lopez M et al. Use of lead-glazed ceramics is the main factor associated to high lead in blood levels in two Mexican rural communities. *Journal of toxicology and environmental health*, 1994, 42(1):45–52.

15. Romieu I et al. Sources of lead exposure in Mexico City. *Environmental health perspectives*, 1994, 102(4):384–389.

16. Hernandez AM. Lead-glazed ceramics as major determinants of blood levels in Mexican women. *Environmental health perspectives*, 1991, 94:117–120.

17. Albert LA, Badillo F. Environmental lead in Mexico. *Reviews of environmental contamination and toxicology*, 1991, 117:1–49.

18. *Survey of lead and cadmium in glazed tableware.* Perth, Health Department of Western Australia, 1995.

19. *FDA Consumer.* Washington, DC, Food and Drug Administration, July/August 1987 (FDA 87-1139).

20. Motarjemi Y et al. Contaminated weaning food: a major risk factor for diarrhoea and associated malnutrition. *Bulletin of the World Health Organization*, 1993, 71(1):79–92.

21. *The role of food safety in health and development. Report of a Joint FAO/WHO Expert Committee on Food Safety.* Geneva, World Health Organization, 1984 (WHO Technical Report Series, No. 705).

22. Beaglehole R, Bonita R, Kjellström T. *Basic epidemiology.* Geneva, World Health Organization, 1993.

23. Kapperud G et al. Risk factors for *Toxoplasma gondii* infection in pregnancy. Results of a prospective case–control study in Norway. *American journal of epidemiology*, 1996, 44(4):405–412.

24. Baltazar JC, Tiglao TV, Tempongko SB. Hygiene behaviour and hospitalized severe childhood diarrhoea: a case–control study. *Bulletin of the World Health Organization*, 1993, 71(3):323–328.

25. Dikassa L et al. Maternal behavioural risk factors for severe childhood diarrhoeal disease in Kinshasa, Zaire. *International journal of epidemiology*, 1993, 22(2):327–333.

26. Daniels DL et al. A case–control study of the impact of improved sanitation on diarrhoea and morbidity in Lesotho. *Bulletin of the World Health Organization*, 1990, 68(4):455–463.

27. Maung K et al. Risk factors for the development of persistent diarrhoea and malnutrition in Burmese children. *International journal of epidemiology*, 1990, 21(5):1021–1029.

28. Echeverria P et al. Case–control study of endemic diarrhea disease in Thai children. *Journal of infectious diseases*, 1989, 159:543–548.

29. Weber JT et al. Epidemic cholera in Ecuador: multidrug resistance and transmission by water and seafood. *Epidemiology and infection*, 1994, 112(1):1–11.

30. Hoge CW et al. Epidemiologic study of *Vibrio cholerae* O1 and O139 in Thailand: at the advancing edge of the eighth pandemic. *American journal of epidemiology*, 1996, 143(3):263–268.

31. Knight SM et al. Risk factors for the transmission of diarrhoea in children: a case control study in rural Malaysia. *International journal of epidemiology*, 1992, 21(4):812–818.

32. Codex Alimentarius Commission. *Food hygiene basic texts.* Rome, Food and Agriculture Organization of the United Nations/World Health Organization, 1997.

33. Lambiri M, Mavridou A, Papdakis JA. The application of Hazard Analysis Critical Control Point (HACCP) in a flight catering establishment improved the bacteriological quality of meals. *Journal of the Royal Society of Health*, 1995 (February):26–30.

34. Bryan FL. *Hazard Analysis Critical Control Point evaluations—a guide to identifying hazards and assessing risks associated with food preparation and storage.* Geneva, World Health Organization, 1992.

35. *Essential safety requirements for street-vended foods.* Geneva, World Health Organization, 1996 (unpublished document WHO/FNU/FOS/96.7; available on request from Food Safety, World Health Organization, 1211 Geneva 27, Switzerland).

36. *Training aspects of the Hazard Analysis Critical System. Report of a WHO workshop on training in HACCP.* Geneva, World Health Organization, 1996 (unpublished document WHO/FNU/FOS/96.3; available on request from Food Safety, World Health Organization, 1211 Geneva 27, Switzerland).

37. Worsfold D, Griffith C. A generic model for evaluating consumer food safety behaviour. *Food control,* 1995, 6(6):357–363.

38. *Application of the Hazard Analysis Critical Control Point system for the improvement of food safety. WHO supported case studies on food prepared in homes, street vending operations, and in cottage industries.* Geneva, World Health Organization, 1993 (unpublished document WHO/FNU/FOS/93.1; available on request from Food Safety, World Health Organization, 1211 Geneva 27, Switzerland).

39. Desmarchelier PM et al. Evaluation of the safety of domestic food preparation in Malaysia. *Bulletin of the World Health Organization,* 1994, 72(6):877–884.

40. Bryan FL et al. Hazards associated with holding and reheating foods at vending sites in small town in Zambia. *Journal of food protection,* 1997, 60(4):391–398.

41. Schmitt R et al. Hazards and critical control points of food preparation in homes in which persons had diarrhea in Zambia. *Journal of food protection,* 1997, 60(2):161–171.

42. Jermini M et al. Hazards associated with holding and reheating foods of food vending operations in a large city in Zambia. *Journal of food protection,* 1997, 60(3):288–299.

43. *Report on street vended and weaning foods in Yangon, Myanmar.* Geneva, World Health Organization, 1995 (unpublished document; available on request from Food Safety, World Health Organization, 1211 Geneva 27, Switzerland).

44. *Education for health: A manual on health education in primary health care.* Geneva, World Health Organization, 1988.

45. Wyatt CJ. Concerns, experiences, attitudes and practices of food market managers regarding sanitation and safe food handling procedures. *Journal of food protection,* 1979, 42(7):555–560.

46. Burch N, Sawyer C. Food handling in convenience stores: the impact of personnel knowledge on facility sanitation. *Journal of environmental health,* 1991, 54(3):23–27.

47. Abidoye RO, Otokiti EA. Environmental and health evaluation of food handlers in Nigerian bukaterias. *Catering and health,* 1990, 1:259–264.

48. Burger J, Staine K, Gochefeld M. Fishing in contaminated waters: knowledge and risk perception of hazards by fishermen in New York City. *Journal of toxicology and environmental health,* 1993(1):95–105.

49. Alterkruse SF et al. Consumer knowledge of foodborne microbial hazards and food-handling practices. *Journal of food protection,* 1996, 59(3):287–294.

50. Klontz KC et al. Prevalence of selected food consumption and preparation behaviours associated with increased risks of foodborne disease. *Journal of food protection,* 1995, 58(8):927–930.

51. Kidevand H, Holm L. Consumers' views on food quality. A qualitative interview study. *Appetite,* 1996, 27:1–14.

52. Oltersdorf U. *Consumer knowledge about aspects of food hygiene and food safety, results of a nationwide survey in Germany.* Paper presented at Food Micro, 15th international symposium, International Committee on Food Microbiology and Hygiene, Bingen, 31 August–3 September 1993 (available on request from Ulrich Oltersdorf, Institute for the Economics and Sociology of Nutrition, Federal Agency for Research in Nutrition, Garbenstrasse 13, D-70599 Stuttgart, Germany).

53. Hodges I. *Raw to cooked food. Community awareness of safe food handling practices.* Wellington, New Zealand Department of Health, 1993.

54. Resurreccion AVA et al. Consumer attitudes toward irradiated food: results of a new study. *Journal of food protection,* 1995, 58(2):193–196.

55. Dawson S, Manderson L, Tallo VL. *A manual for the use of focus groups.* Boston, MA, International Nutrition Foundation for Developing Countries, 1993.

56. *Report of food safety labelling.* Toronto, Ontario Ministry of Agriculture, Food and Rural Affairs, 1996.

57. Teague JL, Anderson DW. Consumer preferences for safe food handling labels on meat and poultry. *Journal of consumer affairs,* 1995, 29(1);108–127.

58. *Participatory hygiene and sanitation transformation. A new approach to working with communities.* Geneva, World Health Organization, 1996 (unpublished document WHO/EOS/96.11; available on request from Department of Protection of the Human Environment, World Health Organization, 1211 Geneva 27, Switzerland).

CHAPTER 4

Strategies and partners

Food safety education programmes should aim to improve the knowledge and practice of policy-makers, food producers, food processors, professional food handlers and consumers as all have a role to play in food safety. However, certain groups, either because of their direct role in food preparation or their greater vulnerability to foodborne diseases, need to receive greater emphasis in the programme.

These include:

— domestic food handlers, particularly mothers of small children;
— professional food handlers, including those who handle, prepare or serve food in cottage industries,[1] food and catering establishments, retail outlets and supermarkets, as well as street food vendors;
— high-risk groups, including travellers.

Governments, and in particular the health sector, have the leading role in health education in food safety. They are responsible for initiating, coordinating and implementing food safety educational programmes and related measures. However, the impact is strengthened if the educational programme is developed and implemented in partnership and collaboration with other sectors or community groups. Examples of partners who are in a position to influence food handlers and consumers, the role that each partner could play, and some examples of initiatives which have been taken in this area are discussed below.

Health sector

Maternal and child health clinics and primary health care centres

The importance of these centres in the prevention of foodborne diseases is considerable. These centres are visited by pregnant women and the mothers of infants and small children who are the primary victims of food contamination and incorrect food safety practices. Therefore, maternal and child health centres can play a tremendously important role in the protection of infants and children by advising pregnant women and mothers in food safety (*1–3*). As mothers are

---

[1] Food handlers working in medium-to-large industries also require training and education in food safety. However, the focus of this book is on those small operations which have received less attention and where formal food control authorities have limited power to control the safety of food.

usually motivated to protect their children they are likely to be receptive to food safety messages.

Pregnant women

There are a number of foodborne infections, notably listeriosis and toxoplasmosis, which may adversely affect the fetus. Chemical contaminants such as lead and methylmercury, depending on their level of intake, may also have negative effects on the health of the fetus. Maternal and child health centres and primary health care centres have the responsibility of informing pregnant women about types of food or practices that may present risks to them and their unborn children.

A number of laudable measures of this nature have been taken in some countries. In Sweden, a poster giving dietary advice on all types of food which may be unsafe, combined with nutritional advice, is distributed to pregnant women through maternal and child health centres. In several other countries (e.g. Australia, France, New Zealand, United Kingdom and USA) brochures are provided at maternal and child health centres on food safety for the prevention of listeriosis (*4–10*). In the United Kingdom, health education material on the prevention of toxoplasmosis is produced for professionals and pregnant women (*11*). In France, a brochure outlining risks of listeriosis and toxoplasmosis, as well as of tobacco and alcohol, is distributed to pregnant women (*10*).

Lactating women

Breast milk is the ideal source of nourishment and the safest food for infants during their first (4–6) months of life. It protects them against foodborne diarrhoea through anti-infective properties and by minimizing exposure to foodborne pathogens. Education of expectant mothers in food safety should include information on breastfeeding. Major efforts are being made at national and international levels to promote breastfeeding, and a great deal of educational material is available for advising mothers on this subject. It is beyond the scope of this book to list the large number of initiatives and extensive material on this subject; thus readers are referred to standard sources for such information (*12–14*).

However, it should be remembered that certain chemical contaminants, particularly fat-soluble contaminants, can pass into human milk. The source of these contaminants can be food consumed by nursing mothers during the breast-feeding period, and particularly the mobilization of body fat in which contaminants have accumulated from previous exposures. Current intake of pharmaceuticals or drug abuse (including tobacco and alcohol), as well as environmental and occupational exposure (which can include dermal and inhalation exposures), can also contribute to the levels of potentially harmful substances in human milk. Therefore, every effort should be made to protect breast milk from such contamination.

Health practitioners are usually aware that certain drugs are contraindicated for breastfeeding mothers. However, the risk of toxic substances in food passing into breast milk is often not considered. The presence of some substances at high levels in human milk has in the past produced adverse health effects in infants. In several instances, where mothers were affected by toxic chemical substances such as hexachlorobenzene, methylmercury and ciguatoxin, the breastfed infants were also affected to varying degrees. In a case of mass intoxication in Iraq in 1972, over 6000 people were affected by the consumption of seed grain treated with methylmercury. Infants exposed through breast milk suffered from severe acute and chronic adverse health effects, including neurological disorders, decreased intelligence and mental retardation (*15*). Cases of ciguatera have also been observed in infants who were exposed to the toxin through breast milk (*16*). Therefore, when lactating mothers are intoxicated or heavily exposed to chemicals, the long-term and short-term risks for infants should be evaluated and proper advice should be provided to the mothers. Such advice may vary with the situation, and can range from dietary guidance in order to minimize the level of contaminants in breast milk to abstinence from breastfeeding in extreme cases. However, any guidance limiting the period of breastfeeding should be carefully considered in light of the significant benefits of breast-feeding and the known risk of foodborne infections due to exposure to foodborne pathogens through alternative feeding (*17*).

Some governments (e.g. Canada, Sweden and several states in the USA) have developed an information strategy advising pregnant or lactating women who are consuming large amounts of freshwater fish to limit their consumption of some fish and to avoid certain types of fish known to be highly contaminated. For example, in a leaflet entitled *Goda raad om fisk* (Good advice about fish) the Swedish Government recommended that women who are pregnant, lactating or plan to become pregnant should limit their consumption of fish of several species and avoid others (*18*). The leaflet was made available to the target group through maternal and child health centres. The Swedish Government has also recommended that nursing women should not lose large amounts of weight abruptly, in order to avoid increasing levels of contaminants in breast milk as these are mobilized from fat stores (*19*). WHO's Regional Office for Europe made a similar recommendation against weight loss (*20*), as have several states in the USA and provinces in Canada (*21*).

In addition to chemical contaminants, there is evidence that the human immunodeficiency virus (HIV)—the virus which causes the acquired immunodeficiency syndrome (AIDS)—can be transmitted through breastfeeding. Various studies conducted to date indicate that between one-quarter and one-third of infants born worldwide to women infected with HIV become infected with the virus themselves. Preliminary studies indicate that about one-third of infected infants are infected through breastfeeding. Therefore, counselling women who are aware of their HIV status should include the best available information on the benefits of breastfeeding as well as on the risk of HIV transmission through breastfeeding, and on the risks and possible advantages associated with other methods of infant feeding. Parents, particularly mothers, should be enabled to make an informed choice. If an alternative feeding method is chosen by the parents, it is essential that mothers are taught to prepare a breast-milk substitute which is safe and nutritionally adequate (*22*). As with chemical contaminants, any advice on limiting or abstaining from breast-feeding should be based on a careful analysis of the risks and benefits of the different feeding alternatives.

Mothers of older infants and young children

While public health authorities have recognized the importance of breast-feeding in the prevention of foodborne diseases, little attention has been paid to the importance of safe food handling during the preparation of complementary foods. The fact that the incidence of diarrhoeal diseases continues to be high—according to some sources, it has not decreased during the last 10 years (*23*)—provides clear evidence that current efforts, which consist mainly of the promotion of breastfeeding, vaccination against childhood diseases and improvement of water supply and sanitation, are far from sufficient and that these efforts should be extended to the improvement of food safety in households.

Many studies have shown that foods prepared in homes under unhygienic conditions are frequently contaminated and are the major cause of diarrhoea and associated malnutrition in infants and young children (*1, 24–35*) (see Box 14). It is estimated that contamination of food may be the cause of up to

---

Box 14. Complementary foods and infant and child diarrhoea

Numerous studies have shown that weaning foods prepared under unhygienic conditions are frequently heavily contaminated with pathogenic agents and are a major risk factor in the transmission of diseases, especially diarrhoeal diseases. Studies by Black et al. in Bangladesh showed that 41% of the samples of food items fed to children of weaning age contained *E. coli*. Milk and foods prepared specially for infants were more frequently and heavily contaminated with *E. coli* than foods prepared for adults such as boiled rice. The level of contamination was also found to be related to the storage of complementary foods at high ambient temperatures. About half of drinking-water samples also contained *E. coli*, but colony counts were approximately 10 times lower than in food samples. A major important finding was the correlation between the proportion of a child's food samples contaminated with *E. coli* and the number of annual episodes of diarrhoea associated with enterotoxigenic *E. coli* (*25, 26*). Bacterial contamination of weaning foods and drinking-water was also studied in rural Bangladesh by Henry et al. (*26*). Some 900 samples of food and drinking-water were analysed for faecal coliforms, and it was found that the so-called "wet" foods (such as milk and rice which make up a large proportion of a child's weaning diet in the 6–23 month age range) contained the highest levels of faecal coliforms, and that during the rainy season when ambient temperatures increased, the level of contamination also increased. The contamination of food with faecal coliforms is an indication that food is contaminated with faecal matter and thus may be a vehicle for pathogens usually transmitted by the faecal–oral route, including *Shigella* spp. and *V. cholerae*.

Similarly, studies conducted in other parts of the world provide evidence of the significant contamination of complementary foods. Barrel et al. found that a very high proportion of the food consumed by infants and young children in a rural area of Gambia contained pathogens. In the rainy and hot season, when diarrhoeal illness is at its height, one-third of the foods were contaminated immediately after their preparation with unacceptable levels of one or more pathogens, and this increased to 96% when the food was stored for eight hours (*27*). In Myanmar, food consumed by children between 6 and 29 months of age was examined for four enteric bacterial pathogens. Of 775 samples of food tested, 505 (65%) were positive for *E. coli*, 28 (3.6%) for *V. cholerae* non-01 and 6 (0.8%) for *Salmonella*. *E. coli* and *V. cholerae* non-01 were isolated from 29 (25.7%) and 5 (4.7%) water samples respectively from a total of 113 drinking-water samples (*28*). In Peru, menu items given to infants were studied at the time of consumption. Milk and food specially prepared for infants (cereals or purées) were most frequently contaminated, whereas foods eaten by an entire family, such as soups, stews and fried foods, were less often contaminated. For most food items, the frequency of contamination was related to the amount of time after initial preparation. Specific pathogens found in food included *Salmonella, Aeromonas hydrophila, V. cholerae* non-01 and enterotoxigenic *E. coli* (*29*). As complementary foods are often selected from items in the adults' diet, the hygienic quality of adult food is also of relevance in this context. HACCP studies conducted in households in the Dominican Republic showed that cooked food products, particularly beans, rice, dried milk, if subjected to time–temperature abuse, contained high amounts of *Bacillus cereus, Staphylococcus aureus* and also faecal coliforms (*30, 31*). In Guatemala, heavy contamination with coliforms, *Bacillus cereus* and staphylococci was found in tortillas before and after cooking (*32*). In El Salvador, 18% of foods were found to be contaminated with *E. coli* (*33*). In an investigation of a large urban epidemic of cholera in Guinea, it was found that peanut sauce supported the growth of *V. cholerae* and was the probable vehicle for transmission of the disease (*34*).

70% of diarrhoeal disease occurring worldwide in infants and children. In view of this it is unquestionable that education of mothers and care-givers in food safety principles is vital if there is to be a substantial improvement in prevention of diarrhoeal diseases in infants and children. In this area, maternal and child health centres as well as primary health care centres irrefutably have the leading role.

Most of these centres already advise mothers on breastfeeding, infant feeding and nutrition, as well as on other aspects of the care of infants and children. These centres could include information on safe food handling practices. They could, for example, adapt WHO's "*Basic principles for the preparation of safe food for infants and young children*" to local conditions and explain them or make them available to mothers (Box 15) (*2, 36*).

Box 15. Basic principles for the preparation of safe food for infants and young children (Source: *36*)

■ *Cook food thoroughly*

Many raw foods, notably poultry, raw milk and vegetables, are very often contaminated with disease-causing organisms. Thorough cooking will kill these organisms. For this purpose all parts of the food must become steaming hot, which means they must reach a minimum temperature of 70 °C.

■ *Avoid storing cooked food*

Prepare food for infants and young children freshly, and give it to them immediately after preparation when it is cool enough to eat. Foods prepared for infants and young children should preferably not be stored at all. If this is impossible, food could be stored only for the next meal, but kept cool (at temperatures below 10 °C) or hot (at temperatures near or above 60 °C). Stored food should be reheated thoroughly. Again, this means that all parts of the food must reach at least 70 °C.

■ *Avoid contact between raw foodstuffs and cooked foods*

Cooked food can become contaminated through even the slightest contact with raw food. This cross-contamination can be direct, as, for example, when raw food comes into contact with cooked food. It can also be indirect and subtle: for example, through hands, flies, utensils or unclean surfaces. Thus, hands should be washed after handling high-risk foods, e.g. poultry. Similarly, utensils used for raw foods should be carefully washed before they are used again for cooked food. The addition of any new ingredients to cooked food may again introduce pathogenic organisms. In this case, food needs to be thoroughly cooked again.

■ *Wash fruits and vegetables*

Fruit and vegetables, particularly if they are given to infants in raw form, must be washed carefully with safe water. If possible, vegetables and fruits should be peeled. In situations when these foods are likely to be heavily contaminated—for example, when untreated waste water is used for irrigation or untreated nightsoil is used for soil fertilization—fruits and vegetables which cannot be peeled should be thoroughly cooked before they are given to infants.

■ *Use safe water*

Safe water is just as important in preparing food for infants and young children as it is for drinking. Water used in preparing food should be boiled, unless the food to which the water is added has subsequently to be cooked (e.g., rice, potatoes). Remember that ice made of unsafe water will also be unsafe.

■ *Wash hands repeatedly*

Wash hands thoroughly before you start preparing or serving food and after every interruption—especially if you have changed the baby, used the toilet, or been in contact with animals. It should be remembered that household animals often harbour germs that can pass from hands to food.

■ *Avoid feeding infants with a bottle*

Use a spoon and cup to give drinks and liquid foods to infants and young children. It is usually difficult to get bottles and teats completely clean. Spoons, cups, dishes and utensils used for preparing and feeding infants should be washed straight after use. This will facilitate their thorough cleaning. If bottles and teats must be used, they should be thoroughly washed and boiled after every use.

■ *Protect foods from insects, rodents and other animals*

Animals frequently carry pathogenic organisms and are potential sources of contamination of food.

■ *Store non-perishable foodstuffs in a safe place*

Keep pesticides, disinfecting agents, or other toxic chemicals in labelled containers and separate from foodstuffs. To protect against rodents and insects, non-perishable foodstuffs should be stored in closed containers. Containers which have previously held toxic chemicals should not be used for storing foodstuffs.

■ *Keep all food preparation premises meticulously clean*

Surfaces used for food preparation must be kept absolutely clean in order to avoid food contamination. Scraps of food and crumbs are potential reservoirs of germs and can attract insects and animals. Garbage should be kept in safe, covered places and be disposed of quickly.

A number of WHO documents underline the need for the integration of food safety into infant feeding programmes and primary health care (*1–3*). Programmes for training health workers have also been initiated in a number of countries to train the trainers of health workers in food safety. For example, a programme to train nutritionists in food safety has begun in Indonesia. This aims to increase their skills in advising the public in food safety. The course is carried out by the Industry Council for Development (a nongovernmental organization representing major food companies), in collaboration with the Southeast Asian Ministers of Education Organization (SEAMEO) and the German Technical Cooperation Agency (GTZ). A training package has also been developed to this end (*37*). A training package for integrating food safety into the primary health care system is being developed (*38*). The WHO books *Teaching for better learning* and *Education for health* complement the food safety training packages with guidance on teaching methodologies and approaches (*39, 40*). Box 16 describes how the Islamic Republic of Iran has integrated food safety into its primary health care system.

Hospitals, clinics, primary health care centres and health practitioners

Information and education

The role of maternal and child health centres is also valid for hospitals, clinics, primary health care centres and health practitioners. However, as these facilities are in contact with the entire population, from children to the elderly, they have a broader responsibility. They are responsible for giving advice to the population in general and high-risk groups in particular. High-risk groups include:

— travellers;
— the elderly;
— those with underlying health problems (e.g. patients with liver disease, cancer, HIV infection, diabetes, and those who have allergic reactions to certain foods or substances added to food products);
— pregnant women.

Travellers may often consult physicians, the infectious disease clinic of a hospital, or other clinics to obtain vaccination and other prophylactic or therapeutic treatment. Advice on prevailing foodborne diseases in certain countries, and foods and drinks likely to be contaminated, could be provided to travellers through these centres. For this purpose, WHO publishes annually *International travel and health* which gives information on prevailing diseases in different parts of the world, vaccination needs, and precautions to be taken with regard to food and drink (*41*). WHO has also issued a leaflet entitled *A guide on safe food for travellers* which provides recommendations to travellers on how to eat safely

---

Box 16. Integration of food safety into the primary health care system in the Islamic Republic of Iran

Providing education on prevailing health problems, and ensuring basic sanitation, proper nutrition, safe food and safe water are among the essential elements of primary health care. Primary health care is the first level of contact of individuals, families and communities with the national health care system, bringing health care as close as possible to where people live and work. It is the first element in a continuing health care process. So far, primary health care systems, particularly in developing countries, have paid scant attention to the problem of food safety.

One of the first countries to take the initiative to integrate food safety into the primary health care system is the Islamic Republic of Iran. The country has a very comprehensive primary health care system. In addition to hospitals and district health centres, the network includes some 14 000 health houses serving about 1500 people each, 2100 rural health centres covering a population of 7500 persons, and about 2000 urban health centres assisting some 12 500 persons. The primary health care network of the Islamic Republic of Iran provides integrated health services to 85% of the rural population and the entire urban population. The remaining 25% of the rural population are covered by mobile health care teams. The country is implementing a pilot project for integrating food safety into the primary health care system. To this end, six districts were selected because a major share of their people are involved in production of foodstuffs, particularly dairy products, which are a major source of brucellosis in these areas. A programme for training the trainers of primary health care workers in food safety is being implemented. In conjunction with this project, a massive health education campaign is carried out through the media to raise the awareness of consumers.

---

and what to do in case of diarrhoea (*42*). A similar leaflet has been prepared on foods which are safe with regard to cholera (*43*).

The elderly constitute a significant and increasing proportion of the general population and of travellers. The elderly must be made aware that the health consequences of foodborne infections may be more serious for them, and that they may be more susceptible than other segments of the population to some foodborne infections such as enterohaemorrhagic *E. coli* infection and listeriosis. They should avoid high-risk foods such as dishes made from raw or undercooked animal products (eggs, meat, milk) or raw seafood.

Similar information should be provided to those with underlying health problems in order that their health condition should not be further jeopardized. In the United States, a brochure distributed through health care centres informs people with immune disorders, liver disease or diabetes of the risk of certain seafood and the required food safety measures (*44–46*).

Great care should also be taken in the preparation of foods for hospital patients, including the newborn when they are not breastfed. Because of various health conditions or treatments, patients may be more vulnerable to foodborne infections. Reports of foodborne disease outbreaks in Europe indicate 1–10% of foodborne disease outbreaks may occur in the hospitals, medical care institutions or homes for the elderly (*47, 48*). Poor hygiene in the preparation of infant formula has been recognized as the cause of several cases of meningitis in newborn infants in Iceland (*49*). Food handlers working in the hospital kitchen need to be trained in safe food handling, and nurses and dietitians should also receive education in food safety.

The standard of cleanliness and hygienic practice in health care centres sets an example for visitors. A poor standard of hygiene in these places will have a negative effect on people's perception of the importance of hygiene.

Surveillance

Epidemiological data on foodborne illnesses are important for planning and evaluating educational activities, as well as for detecting and controlling outbreaks of foodborne disease. Thus, in addition to advising the public, health care centres should actively participate in the surveillance of foodborne diseases and collaborate with food control authorities by providing information on the incidence and outbreaks of foodborne diseases, and their possible sources. Unfortunately, in many countries the communication channel between different authorities or agencies is weak.

Universities and schools of medicine, nursing and public health

One of the main constraints in food safety is the lack of knowledge or awareness of health workers. Not infrequently, health professionals are not up to date with the epidemiology of certain diseases, and may ignore the foodborne routes of diseases such as cholera, shigellosis and other diarrhoeal diseases. As a consequence, they are not in a position to inform patients and the general public. In a survey of 19 items of health education material for either health workers or the public on the prevention of toxoplasmosis, it was observed that none provided satisfactory information with regard to the source of infection and preventive actions (*11*). It is not uncommon for some foodborne diseases to be misdiagnosed. Moreover, as international travel and trade in food increase, physicians and health workers may be confronted with foodborne diseases that normally occur in other parts of the world and are therefore unknown to them.

For the health sector to fulfil its role with regard to the prevention of foodborne illnesses, it is essential that health workers of all categories, including physicians, nurses and midwives, are better trained in food safety and in the epidemiology of foodborne diseases and are kept abreast of developments.

Universities and colleges providing education and training for these groups of professionals should consider introducing food safety into the curriculum and updating existing programmes with the most recent scientific findings.

Universities and research institutes are also an asset in terms of information on the pathogenicity/toxicity of microorganisms and contaminants, and on underlying factors leading to the increased susceptibility of certain individuals. Their scientific findings are essential for understanding the epidemiology/ etiology of foodborne diseases and for formulating appropriate education approaches.

Education sector

Primary and secondary schools

Schoolchildren are both a target group for education and a channel for educating others.

As a future adult, a child is a potential food handler and may also be a future policy-maker. Healthy habits ingrained in the early years will be applied throughout life.

Many food-related practices are cultural habits, and changes in them are more effectively achieved in the early years of life. Teachers can have a powerful impact by encouraging such change. Furthermore, absenteeism from the school can be a mechanism for surveillance of foodborne diseases.

Schoolchildren are an effective channel for communicating food safety messages to parents or other children. Parents or children may sometimes be more likely to accept such messages from their friends or family members than from outsiders.

Children are themselves often the victims of foodborne diseases from foods prepared in their homes or in school canteens, or bought from street food vendors.[1] Several outbreaks of foodborne intoxications due to the consumption of street food and involving hundreds of children have been reported from African countries. In 1990, an outbreak of foodborne intoxication affected some 200 schoolchildren in Côte d'Ivoire; the outbreak was one of a series of mass intoxications that occurred among schoolchildren in this country (*50*) (see also Table 11).

Schoolchildren are also sometimes victims of the food they prepare themselves in the school during cookery classes. Outbreaks of campylobacteriosis,

---

[1] Food handlers in school canteens represent another category of personnel that must be educated and trained, as many foodborne diseases occur in such environments as a result of mishandling food, and these staff and their actions serve as examples for schoolchildren.

enterohaemorrhagic *E. coli* infections or salmonellosis in schoolchildren who drank raw milk during class visits to farms have occasionally been reported in industrialized countries. A survey of milkborne campylobacteriosis in the USA showed that 35% of outbreaks occurring during a three-year period (1987–1990) were associated with school field trips or other outings (*51*).

Another reason for the need to focus on children is that in many countries older children may take care of their younger siblings when mothers are away from the home at work. Older children may prepare food or feed infants or small children.

Mothers and other food handlers should be discouraged from preparing food when they are suffering from infections with symptoms of diarrhoea, vomiting, fever, sore throat with fever, discharge from the ear, eye or nose, jaundice or skin lesions. Mothers should, if at all possible, delegate this task to other members of the family such as older children. If this is not possible, mothers and other food handlers should be advised to observe strict personal hygiene. Skin lesions should be covered.

The teacher–child–parent approach has been used in a number of countries for health education purposes. In the Philippines, an attempt is being made to integrate food safety into this approach to enhance safe food handling in the home (*52*). Child-to-child education is also an effective means of disseminating information between children in and out of school. Children and adolescents are highly influenced by their peers. The child-to-child approach is being successfully used in some 70 countries in a number of health areas (including nutrition, and prevention of diarrhoea through safe water supply and sanitation) (*52–55*). Regrettably, few countries have applied this approach to education in food safety. In Zambia, the child-to-child approach is being used for the prevention of cholera.

The earlier the training and education start the easier it is to influence behaviour. Therefore, even at kindergarten children should be taught basic rules of food hygiene beginning, for instance, with teaching about washing hands before touching food.

Teacher training colleges

One of the main constraints in teaching food safety to schoolchildren is that the teachers themselves have no education in the subject and often lack teaching materials. To improve education in food safety in school settings, teachers—especially those teaching home economics or related topics—should receive formal training in food safety. Thus, food safety should be integrated into teacher training curricula.

To help train primary school teachers, WHO has developed a guide entitled *Food, environment and health.* This covers food safety and related issues such as housing, sanitation and nutrition (*56*). A teacher's resource book that includes sections on food safety has been prepared by WHO's Regional Offices for Africa and the Eastern Mediterranean in collaboration with UNICEF, UNESCO and the Islamic Educational Scientific and Cultural Organization (ISESCO) (*57*). Guidelines for developing comprehensive school health education have been drawn up jointly by WHO, UNESCO and UNICEF (*58*). A European guide to nutrition education in schools, including food safety considerations, is in preparation (*59*).

At the national level, the United Kingdom Ministry of Agriculture, Fisheries and Food has developed an educational package containing a wallchart, posters, stickers and a 6-minute animated video designed to teach the basic elements of hygiene to primary school children of 5–12 years (*60*). Also in the United Kingdom, *Working with food in primary schools* is a teachers' resource book on food hygiene and safety (*61*). Similarly in New Zealand, a teaching package that includes a video film has been produced for use in secondary schools to reinforce education in food safety (*62*). In Peru, a calendar has been produced that features a different food safety theme for each month (*63*). In countries such as Kenya, Nepal and Peru, comics have been used to explain food safety and nutrition to schoolchildren (*64, 65*).

Universities, colleges and research and training institutions

The expertise of scientists is of immense value to regulatory agencies and food industries in ensuring food safety. Food scientists in particular have the responsibility to understand consumers' fears about new processes and new food products, and to address their concerns. Consumers should be provided with evidence of the benefits and safety of new processes and products for they may otherwise reject innovations in food science and technology. Scientists can help to demystify the sometimes inaccurate perceptions that consumers, and even some public health authorities, have of food technologies (*66–68*).

The collaboration of academic institutions with government, industries and other interested parties in training and education in food safety can be very helpful, particularly if it involves experts in training. An example of such collaboration is provided by the Cooperative Extension of the University of Massachusetts which, in collaboration with the United States Department of Agriculture, developed a half-day training programme for professional food handlers entitled *Food-handling is a risky business*. The Michigan State University Extension has developed a multimedia package for teaching food safety to children (*69*).

Food science is a relatively new science, and there is still a tremendous need for research on processing technologies which may enhance the safety of food. Universities, colleges and research and training institutions should therefore pay greater attention to present problems in food supply and give high priority to research in food safety (*70, 71*).

Tourism sector

As lifestyles change, an increasing number of people eat outside the home in restaurants, on aircraft, on cruise ships, in canteens, at street food vending stands, in camps and so on. For many people, food prepared in these places constitutes an important part of the diet and therefore also a notable source of foodborne disease.

The tourism sector (hotels and restaurants and their associations, catering establishments including airline and cruise ship catering, tour operators, travel agencies, organizers of large fairs and sporting or social events) can play a two-fold role in the prevention of foodborne diseases. They can provide information for travellers to enable them to make wise choices regarding foods in holiday locations and they can actively promote food safety standards in those locations by training food handlers in the essential elements of food safety.

Training and education of professional food handlers

Professional food handlers are responsible for the safe preparation of food for consumers, just as a driver, pilot or captain is responsible for the safety of passengers. Food handlers' education and training are therefore essential. The primary responsibility for such training lies with the manager or proprietor of the food business. The manager must ensure that only trained food handlers are given the responsibility of preparing food. Where necessary, the manager should arrange for appropriate training of employees before they are given the task of preparing food for people or serving it.

Owners and managers of food service and catering establishments should themselves have a thorough knowledge of the management of food hygiene and therefore their education is equally important and should be considered a priority (*72, 73*). A study in Canada showed that restaurants where both managers and food handlers had received education in food safety had higher merit scores when inspected than did restaurants where this was not the case. When only the food handlers had received such education, the restaurants had a better score only for avoiding time–temperature violations (*72*).

Initiatives that the tourism sector can take include integrating food safety into the curricula of hotelier schools and ensuring that continuing education is adequate. This approach would provide systematic training for at least some tourism professionals. However, many food handlers and servers do not attend such schools yet specific education and training should be provided for them. Even when food handlers are recruited on a temporary basis to serve at a large fair, sporting event or social gathering—and particularly in circumstances of mass feeding in emergency situations—care should be taken that these food handlers are trained in essential food safety requirements and that they work under adequate supervision. The importance of training personnel in mass catering cannot be stressed enough since a minor error in food handling may jeopardize the health and life of a large number of people.

Food handlers should receive training in two aspects of food safety—the principles of good hygienic practice and the HACCP system.

The principles of good hygienic practice comprise general know-how on food safety and the basic rules that food handlers should observe. A number of educational and training manuals have been developed in this regard. As examples, a WHO publication provides guidance on hygienic handling of foods (*74*) and a leaflet on hygiene in mass catering has been developed jointly by WHO and Germany's Federal Institute for the Protection of Consumer Health and for Veterinary Medicine (*75*). Specific recommendations on food safety measures for handling eggs and products containing eggs, and on vaccination of food handlers against hepatitis A, have also been developed (*76, 77*). In the framework of the FAO/WHO Codex Alimentarius Commission, a code of hygienic practice for precooked and cooked foods in mass catering is available (*78*). Recommendations have also been developed regarding health surveillance and management procedures for food handlers (*73*) (see also Box 17).

Box 17. WHO recommendations on health surveillance and management procedures for food-handling personnel (*73, 75, 76*)

If suffering from an illness involving *jaundice, diarrhoea, vomiting, fever, sore throat with fever, discharge from ear, eye and nose, visibly infected skin lesions (such as boils, cuts)*, a food handler should report to his or her supervisor. The supervisor should then use discretion as to whether or not the person should be subjected to certain restrictions or suspended from food-handling duties.

Medical advice may be necessary in making this decision. Employees suffering from certain diseases such as typhoid fever or cholera must be cleared medically before being allowed to resume work that involves food handling.

It is recommended that food handlers should not be penalized financially for declaring that they are suffering from an illness or condition that may present a danger to food. Otherwise they may not admit their condition, causing a high risk to consumers and the food business.

Pre-employment or routine medical and laboratory examinations of food-handling personnel are not recommended. Instead, resources should be directed towards education and training.

Vaccination of food handlers against hepatitis A should be considered if resources are available.

The HACCP system is primarily used for assuring safety of foods processed and manufactured in large food industries but WHO has shown that it can be equally applied to the preparation of food in food service establishments, by street food vendors, and in homes (*79*). This is explained in the WHO publication entitled *Hazard Analysis Critical Control Point evaluations: a guide to identifying hazards and assessing risks associated with food preparation and storage* (*80*) (see also Chapter 3). A HACCP training programme for food handlers is being developed, a curriculum for training food inspectors has been drawn up, and training schemes for personnel in large, medium and small industries have been planned (*81*). Application of the HACCP system to mass catering in emergencies and disasters has also been addressed by WHO, UNHCR and the International Federation of Red Cross and Red Crescent Societies (*82*).

The value of training food handlers in HACCP lies in the fact that the food handlers learn to think critically and analytically about the ingredients (including water), the product, the equipment, the process of food preparation and the hazards involved. They learn to identify potential hazards and the control measures that are appropriate to specific operations and circumstances. They also learn to prioritize the control measures, to ensure that those that are critical are applied correctly and meet the necessary conditions, and to take appropriate actions when the conditions are not met.

In mass catering, where thousands of meals are prepared per day, an error in food handling may have catastrophic consequences. The HACCP approach to mass catering provides greater food safety assurance and overcomes constraints such as the high cost of end-product testing and the long delay before results are obtained.

Numerous materials have been developed at national level to support the training of food handlers in the hygienic handling of food and the application of HACCP. Video films have also been developed to help training in safe food handling in various countries. WHO and the Industry Council for Development (ICD) have jointly prepared an inventory of audiovisual material available in food safety and HACCP (*83*).

An important initiative which merits mention as an example of recommended measures for large social events is the training and education of food handlers at the Seville EXPO, in Seville, Spain, in 1992 (Box 18) (*84*).

In some countries, measures have been taken to train professional food handlers and numerous training courses and training materials have been developed (*85–89*). In the United Kingdom, for instance, large numbers of food handlers were trained in basic food hygiene between 1989 and 1995 (*90*). In other countries, as recommended by WHO, pre-employment or routine medical and laboratory examinations of food-handling personnel have been replaced by requirements for the training and education of professional food handlers. A European Union directive stipulates that "food business operators shall

Box 18. Training of food handlers at the Seville EXPO in 1992 (*84*)

This exhibition was held from April to October 1992 on a large island site adjoining the city of Seville. For six months, an average of 200 000 people per day, rising to 500 000 per day at peak periods, visited the 55 000 separate events of EXPO. On the site, visitors were fed at 104 restaurants, 21 cafeterias, 23 bars, 124 kiosks, 150 vending carts and 11 support units, in ambient temperatures rising to 40 °C. A "Health EXPO" unit was responsible for the health and food safety implications of the food operations. Two medical and 25 food control officers supervised the food safety and hygiene. The food safety strategy was based on the application of the HACCP principles, both in regard to the standards which the managers and food handlers had to apply within premises and the points checked by the food control officers who inspected each of the premises at least once every 15 days. The control operation was supported by an epidemiological and health surveillance team and by laboratories that were ready to investigate any reports of foodborne illnesss arising from foods consumed at EXPO and to examine any foods subject to complaints.

The key to the success of the operation was a 15-hour training course for accredited food handlers on the site. This course was given to some 8000 food handlers (including reserve staff) prior to the opening of EXPO. Proprietors and managers of all the EXPO food outlets were provided with a checklist of controls which indicated points to be checked at each stage of food preparation. The same list was used by the inspectors.

In each establishment, 6–8 control points selected from the checklist were identified as critical for minimizing health risks. These included temperature of cooking and storage, cleaning and disinfection, shelving and spacing, and staff health and hygiene. Once the critical control points were identified, the person in charge of the establishment was asked to monitor them carefully by checking certain criteria. Where applicable, a record or register of these checks was kept for examination by the inspector.

This project was developed and implemented by the Spanish Ministry of Health, the Andalusian Health Department and the Seville City Council, in collaboration with the WHO Regional Office for Europe and the Pan American Health Organization. A final analysis of all data collected was carried out in November 1992, and the success of the HACCP approach in the prevention of foodborne disease outbreaks was confirmed. Despite heavy use of all the catering facilities from 9 o'clock in the morning until 4 o'clock in the afternoon every day, no significant report of foodborne illness was received. In particular, there were no reports of illness associated with the consumption of eggs and egg products, despite the fact that in 1992 *Salmonella enteritidis* associated with eggs was a substantial cause of foodborne disease in Spain and the Iberian peninsula.

ensure that food handlers are supervised and instructed and/or trained in food hygiene matters commensurate with their work activity" (*91*).

It has been debated whether training programmes should be mandatory or voluntary. Studies in the USA indicate that voluntary programmes have not been very effective and have attracted mainly the persons who were already committed to food safety rather than those who need the training most. On the other hand, where certification is mandatory there has been clear improvement in the post-training inspection scores (*92*).

For training and educational activities to be effective in ensuring safety, the quality and standard of training are crucial. A poor, or poorly adapted, training programme may be ineffective and may be demoralizing (*92, 93*). Public health authorities should provide guidance regarding training requirements, and should monitor and evaluate training activities. They should also adapt training programmes to the cultural and socioeconomic situation in order not only to change the knowledge and attitudes of food handlers but also to ensure that these are translated into behavioural change and positive actions (*92–94*). At the end of the training course, the competence of food handlers in safe food handling needs to be tested. Certifying food handlers who have successfully passed an examination and achieved a minimum standard of knowledge and skills can stimulate their pride and reinforce the educational messages (*89*). In the United Kingdom, a number of institutions have developed schemes for training and certifying food handlers and managers.

Information and education for travellers

Travel agencies, tour operators, airlines and other transport companies can play an important role in the education of travellers by providing information about high-risk foods and advice about selecting food. To this end, WHO's *Guide on safe food for travellers* can be adapted to local situations (*95*). A number of countries have integrated such food safety advice into their guides for travellers. In the United Kingdom, tour operators have developed a practical manual on *Hygiene and safety in package holidays*. In Sweden, pharmacies distribute a guide which contains extensive food safety advice (*96*).

To raise awareness of the importance of food safety in promoting tourism, the World Tourism Organization and WHO, in collaboration with the national authorities of Mexico and Tunisia, organized three major regional conferences on food safety and tourism. These conferences outlined the role the tourism sector can play in food safety (*97–99*). In Tunisia, the Ministry of Tourism is vigilantly controlling food service establishments to ensure safe food handling and is monitoring the incidence of diarrhoea in travellers to evaluate the impact of food safety measures (*97*).

Food and health inspectors

Food and health inspectors have a pivotal role in food safety. They may represent health, agriculture or tourism departments, as well as municipalities. The role of municipalities in food and health inspection needs to be stressed as in many countries municipal authorities are responsible for the food safety of an ever-increasing urban population.

Inspectors should inspect food services, food retailers and street food vendors, should enforce regulations and should promote the HACCP-based approach to food hygiene. They should also provide educational and advisory services. Frequent inspection of restaurants, although not sufficient by itself, positively influences food-handling practices in these places.

In developing countries, this latter aspect is important. Visits by food and health inspectors may be the only opportunity for food handlers, retailers or street food vendors to receive education in food safety. Food and health inspectors may additionally provide training programmes for specific target groups. The role of inspectors with regard to street food vendors is particularly important. Guidance for training street food vendors is provided in several WHO and FAO documents (*81, 100, 101*).

Food and health inspectors may also assist medical and epidemiological staff in the investigation of foodborne disease outbreaks. They may participate in informing and educating consumers by setting up bureaux dealing with consumer queries and complaints. They can initiate or participate in the development of educational material for consumers and food handlers. Their experience in terms of errors in food handling, and the queries and complaints of consumers, is valuable and should be integrated into education and training programmes.

In times of emergencies and disasters, environmental conditions deteriorate. Lifeline services (electric power, water, sanitation) are often disrupted, and if large numbers of displaced persons gather in one place, the overload on waste disposal systems may increase the risk of foodborne diseases. Food and health inspectors have a vital role in informing the public how to cope with such conditions and in ensuring that temporary food handlers working in mass feeding centres observe the rules of food hygiene (*72*).

Mass media

Media, including radio, television, newspapers, magazines and other types of printed matter, are a major source of information on topical issues and have a tremendous influence in moulding public opinion. Mass media can also play a key role in creating public awareness of food safety issues. As a vehicle for advertising, the media can bring messages into every home, repeatedly and with varying degrees of subtlety. Where governments wish to disseminate health messages, the use of the media although often expensive has maximum effect. In circumstances where resources are limited, use of the media can be limited to reinforcement of other means of communication. In times of emergencies, epidemics, outbreaks or natural disasters, use of the media to disseminate urgent health messages should be regarded as a high priority.

There are dangers that fears about food safety may be enhanced by inaccurate or inadequate information by mass media. It is therefore essential that the health authorities are constantly in touch with the media and give a fair and accurate assessment of problems so that reliable and appropriate messages go out to the public. As demonstrated by the public information campaign during the outbreak of *E. coli* in the United Kingdom (Box 19), it is also important that public health authorities do not rely only on what the mass media tell the public but actively make announcements in the newspapers or on television or radio to inform people of measures to prevent foodborne diseases. Such public information should be given not only in response to crisis but on a regular basis (*102*).

Box 19. Public information during an outbreak

In November 1996, central Scotland in the United Kingdom experienced an outbreak of *E. coli* 0157 infection. This was a serious outbreak causing 19 deaths and 496 cases. In the early stage of the outbreak, a link was established between the infection and consumption of cooked meat products from a butcher. It was therefore decided to inform the public by publicizing details of the suspected contaminated food. The purpose of this was:

- to inform people about the suspected contaminated meat so that they could avoid exposure;
- to inform them what they should do if they had already been exposed to the meat and had developed certain symptoms;
- to give them accurate information about *E. coli* 0157 and how to prevent its transmission.

Initially, a daily press release about the outbreak was issued by the local health authority. The press release contained information about the number of people affected, the suspected source and mode of transmission, as well as information on food and personal hygiene. However, after monitoring what was written in newspapers, it became clear that most of the public health messages in the press release did not appear in the press. The main emphasis of the press was critical rather than informative. The spotlight consistently focused on those individuals or organizations perceived to have failed in their responsibilities to protect the public health.

As a result of this analysis of media coverage, additional methods were adopted to relay the public health message to the community. These included:

- putting announcements in the newspapers about 10 fundamental infection control procedures that people could adopt at home, and at places of work and recreation;
- producing leaflets with the same information and distributing them to every household in the area affected by the outbreak;
- setting up a free telephone line so that people could phone for advice and reassurance;
- giving television and radio interviews;
- setting up a clinic in the middle of the town affected by the outbreak where people could consult a health care worker for counselling, investigation and treatment.

These approaches proved very successful and an evaluation after the outbreak showed that over 95% of the local population had seen, heard or been aware of the public health messages from the health authority (*104*).

Source: Personal communication from S. Ahmed, Consultant in Public Health Medicine, Hamilton, United Kingdom.

Different types of radio and television programme can be used to communicate food safety to the public. News, drama programmes and public service announcements can all deal with food safety issues. Even quiz programmes can include questions on food safety. Cookery programmes can demonstrate the principles of safe food handling. Radio, television and videos are particularly important in explaining food safety to persons who do not read (*103, 104*).

Newspapers can be used to inform the public on food safety issues and remind them about simple food safety measures. Box 20 presents an example from Zimbabwe, where newspapers have been used regularly to remind the public of measures to control and prevent cholera. In Guatemala, a major newspaper devoted an entire page every month to publishing a calendar with food safety messages.

Comics are particularly attractive to children and adolescents and can be used effectively for the education of this target group. Examples are *Pied crow*, a Kenyan children's comic on environment which devoted one issue to food and health (*64*), and *Haamro Sathi* (Our friend) in Nepal which devoted its first issue to water safety (*65*).

A collection of examples of printed food safety educational material produced in different countries has been issued by WHO (*63*). In Guatemala, for instance, a flip chart has been produced containing food safety messages for the prevention of cholera and other foodborne diseases that are prevalent

---

Box 20. Cholera prevention announcement in the press in Zimbabwe, 1993

Cholera alert

There are no reported cases of cholera in Zimbabwe, but there are reports of cholera cases in the neighbouring countries. Therefore, people in Zimbabwe need to be vigilant on the possibility of cholera spreading in the country. In view of the situation, travellers and refugees from affected countries are likely to spread cholera. Prevent cholera by supporting the Government efforts in your area.

Cholera can be spread through
– person eating contaminated and poorly cooked food
– drinking contaminated water
– poor hygienic conditions
– fruits which are not washed and eaten

To prevent cholera, ensure
Practise good hygiene:

– washing hands before handling food
– washing all fruits and vegetables before eating
– boiling all drinking water from unprotected sources
– reheat food before eating
– cover all foods before and after eating
– proper use of toilets at all times
– washing hands with soap and water after using the toilets

Report any severe cases of diarrhoea and vomiting in a person older than 10 years or an increase in the daily number of cases of diarrhoea and vomiting, especially those with watery stools, to the nearest Health Centre, Clinic, Hospital or Doctor.

FOR FURTHER INFORMATION PLEASE CONTACT YOUR NEAREST HEALTH WORKER OR HEALTH FACILITY

Let us prevent cholera!!
PRODUCED BY HEALTH EDUCATION UNIT IN COLLABORATION WITH EPIDEMIOLOGY AND DISEASE CONTROL UNIT, MINISTRY OF HEALTH.

---

in the country (e.g. cysticercosis). The Austrian Government circulated a document containing detailed information on food safety rules to all households (*105*). Similar documents have also been produced in Australia, Germany, Singapore, United Kingdom, USA and elsewhere (*106–131*). Information in printed form may often be referred to in magazines and journals, thus reaching an even wider readership.

Box 21. Playing cards provide education in food safety

In Finland, playing cards have been produced to educate people in food safety while they play. Each of the 52 cards and 2 jokers has one important food safety message (in black) and one piece of advice (in red) printed on them. Each of the four suits represents a different area of food safety. Hearts represent labelling, clubs represent food handling, spades represent food additives and diamonds represent microbiology and pesticides. For example, the ten of diamonds gives the following information: "Uncooked chicken can contain salmonella; cook it thoroughly and wash hands and all tools used after handling."

Other innovative ways of communicating food safety have included drama, telephone hotlines, songs and games (Box 21). The Internet is also a very efficient way of disseminating information to the general public.

The food industry

The food industry—from primary, processing and manufacturing plants to mass catering and food service establishments—is responsible for the safety of the food it offers to the public. To this end, the industry should see that all its employees, from the highest level of management to temporary food handlers or serving personnel, receive appropriate education and training in food safety. The strongest incentive for the food industry to educate employees in food safety is consumer response, i.e. the unwillingness of the consumer to buy food from premises that are unhygienic or that have a bad reputation for food safety. A foodborne disease outbreak that occurs as a result of errors in food processing or food handling will have tremendous economic consequences for the industry.

However, the role of the food industry goes beyond education and training of employees. It extends to the education of consumers in the safe use of products, whether raw, semi-processed or ready-to-eat food. It is in the direct interest of the manufacturer to ensure that all consumers—irrespective of their level of literacy and ability to read labels—are effectively educated in food safety and are able to appreciate real food safety risks. Otherwise, the food industry may wrongly be blamed for food contamination and subsequent illness which result from mishandling of foods by consumers (*132*). The importance of the collaboration of the health sector with industry has been acknowledged in the Declaration of Alma-Ata regarding primary health care which calls for coordinated efforts of various sectors. In addition to the health sector, it refers to agriculture, animal husbandry, food and industry (*133*). Box 22 describes an initiative to promote safe food handling in the United Kingdom.

Education of consumers may occur as a result of consumers' requests for information or as a result of complaints. As in other industries, the food industry could use labels or packaging to convey food safety information to consumers. Alternatively, an information sheet could be inserted into the package.

Box 22. Initiative taken in the United Kingdom to promote safe food handling in the community

In the United Kingdom, the Chartered Institute of Environmental Health and the Food and Drink Federation jointly initiated a food safety campaign, *The Foodlink Campaign and National Food Safety Week*, to promote the concept of shared responsibility in the community, including producers, manufacturers, distributors, retailers and consumers. The initiative consists of a survey of knowledge and understanding of issues relating to food handling and incidence of foodborne diseases, and a food safety education campaign targeted at women aged 25–40 who are the principal food preparers in the home. The campaign includes the distribution of a booklet entitled *Foodlink: A-Z of food safety*, containing 26 food safety messages, through some 400 local authorities, hundreds of consumer groups and voluntary bodies, schools, food and drink manufacturers, retailers, health professionals and the media. During National Food Safety Week, some 400 000 booklets and 3 million information cards were distributed. Some 20 000 posters and 10 000 display cards promoted the "Foodlink" messages. Hundreds of events and activities, including display presentations, competitions entitled "hazard kitchens", media competitions and broadcasts, were held throughout the country, with nine major retailers and many smaller ones being involved.

In most countries, information currently provided on labels relates mainly to the product itself (e.g. quantity, manufacturer and nutritional value). Generally, the food safety related information is very limited and often consists of mandatory information such as information on the shelf-life of the product (e.g. the "use by" date) and, for some products, storage requirements (*134*). In Canada, for instance, the Food and Drug Act and Regulations require the following information on the labels of packaged food: a list of ingredients, the net quantity, the name and address of the manufacturer or importer, and the common name of the food. Labels of products with a durable life of 90 days or less must indicate the expiry date of the durable life with "best before" somewhere on the label. Instructions for proper storage, if they differ from normal room temperature, must also be on the label. In the USA, the trend is towards more detailed labelling requirements. Since July 1994, the US Department of Agriculture has required safe food handling information on all packages of raw and partially cooked meat and poultry products. The labels are described in the Code of Federal Regulations, title 9, parts 317 and 381 (*134*). The label consists of icon and text and states:

This product was prepared from inspected and passed meat and/or poultry. Some food products may contain bacteria that could cause illness if the product is mishandled or cooked improperly. For your protection, follow these safe handling instructions.

Parts of the food industry have voluntarily taken steps to inform consumers about the proper handling of food. In Switzerland, a supermarket chain provides instructions on safe handling of poultry on the label inside the package as well as on handouts to consumers. In Pakistan, WHO's *Ten golden rules for safe food preparation* are displayed on the back of a cornflakes package.

An initiative by major British retail companies involves the establishment of an independent scientific group, the Food Safety Advisory Centre, to provide factual information on food safety to the public. This group produces information leaflets and has established a toll-free telephone number so that consumers can ask questions about food safety (*135*).

Food companies, trade associations and other bodies in industrialized countries distribute various educational materials on aspects of food and nutrition, including food safety. The International Life Sciences Institute (ILSI) supports research, updating scientific facts and raising awareness through conferences and publications. This publication was developed with the support of ILSI.

The Industry Council for Development makes the expertise of the food industry available to governments, other industries and development agencies. ICD has collaborated with WHO in a number of projects, including training courses, seminars, HACCP studies, and the production of educational material and publications.

At the initiative of leading food and beverage companies, the European Food Information Council (EUFIC) has been formed to provide factual and science-based information in the areas of health and nutrition, safety and quality, and the application of modern biotechnology in food. EUFIC has a similar mandate to the International Food Information Council (IFIC) which focuses mostly on the United States market (*136*). For instance, EUFIC undertook a pan-European survey to better understand the views and practices of schoolchildren in different European countries on food safety and nutrition (*137*).

Food industries can play a unique role in the health education of consumers through social marketing. This involves using a systematic methodology adapted from commercial marketing so that a social objective involving a change in behaviour in a specific population group can be achieved. Social marketing can be used by industries to change behaviour by promoting a specific product (*138*). In a number of health areas (e.g. oral health and the prevention of AIDS), companies' advertisements have been very helpful in changing people's attitudes and habits. Advertisements for toothpaste have promoted oral hygiene, and advertisements for condoms have contributed to the prevention of the spread of AIDS. This approach to health education has not yet been fully exploited within the food or related industries. For example, soap could be advertised for its role in removing microorganisms, rather than for softening the skin; and refrigerators could be advertised for their importance in controlling foodborne bacteria and their efficiency in cooling which is essential for proper storage of food. Checking of storage temperature could be promoted by the manufacturers of thermometers. Unfortunately, the advertisements used by some food companies have sometimes seriously misinformed consumers about food safety. For example, some manufacturers have advertised the fact that their products are free from food additives and as a consequence have conveyed the idea that food additives are detrimental to health.

In the Islamic Republic of Iran, the population is reminded of the possible microbial contamination of raw fruits and vegetables by manufacturers of disinfectant agents. In Trinidad and Tobago, collaboration of a number of companies with the health authorities has been effective in preventing cholera (Box 23) (*138*). An example of how grocery distributors in Canada supported a food safety campaign is described in Box 24.

The community

Finally, the whole community should participate in health education in food safety to make sure that food and water are produced and stored in a clean environment, and processed and handled hygienically. Only through the concerted efforts of the whole community can an improvement in food safety standards reasonably be expected.

The role of some groups in the community is particularly important.

Consumer groups and other nongovernmental organizations

A number of organizations represent consumers and defend their rights and interests vis-à-vis governments, industries and other institutions. Some advise consumers on matters related to their health. In this position, they have the unique opportunity to participate in consumer education on food safety. They can raise the consumers' awareness of food safety concerns, stress the need for consumers and

---

Box 23. Collaboration of industry and public health authorities in prevention of cholera in Trinidad and Tobago (*138*)

During the first half of 1992 the threat of cholera in Trinidad and Tobago prompted a strong health education effort by public health authorities and the private sector.

The private sector was mobilized to support government efforts by sponsoring advertisements and announcements in two leading journals to keep cholera prevention in the public eye. A sum of US$ 94 000 was spent by various companies—including bleach and soap companies, cleaning and refuse collection companies, food and beverage processing companies, insurance companies, plastic companies, supermarkets and water treatment companies. The contribution of the private sector to the prevention of cholera was publicly recognized by the Ministry of Health.

Box 24. Canadian grocery distributors support food safety campaign

The Canadian Council of Grocery Distributors (CCGD), consisting of chains of small and large supermarkets, decided to actively promote food safety in homes. Radio was chosen as the medium for communication since messages on radio would be received by the 38% of the population that is functionally illiterate, as well as by those who read regularly.

In collaboration with the Ministry of Health, 16 30-second radio messages were produced for different seasons of the year. The cost of their development, production and distribution was covered by CCGD, with contributions from five commodity groups in exchange for a mention made at the end of the message about their commodities. In January 1996, 108 radio stations across Canada (80 English and 28 French) started to broadcast the messages which were specific to the time of year and associated food safety problems. The content of the messages varied and included information on symptoms of foodborne illnesses, risks associated with eggs, hamburgers, storage of food, and measures for ensuring food safety.

The messages were public service announcements which are broadcast free of charge. As CCGD is a non-profit association, it qualified to use public service announcements.

To complement the radio campaign, similar messages were printed and sent to 178 newspapers and magazines, with a request that they participate in this important public awareness effort. The media were instructed to direct enquiries to health authorities.

CCGD's members were urged to support this initiative by educating their employees and customers. They were provided with the English and French texts of the food safety messages and advised to use them in the same seasonal rhythm as the radio. It was recommended that the messages be included in weekly circulars, or given out with grocery bags. Provincial health ministries offered their toll-free numbers and expertise.

Source: Personal contribution by M. Simon, Canadian Council of Grocery Distributors, 1996.

---

food handlers to observe the rules for safe food preparation in their homes and advise them to be discriminating in their choice of food.

They can also play an important role in raising the awareness of policy-makers for better surveillance and control of safety. They could collaborate with governments and industries in disseminating information to consumers.

Local, grass-roots organizations and women's groups are ideally suited to effect food safety changes in their communities. They are aware of cultural constraints, they speak the language and they know best how to get their message through. Providing them with user-friendly guidelines and information encourages them to take action. Women's associations should be particularly sensitive to the dilemmas of mothers who have small children and who work outside the home, and how this affects their infant feeding. In developing countries, lack of time has often been an impediment for working women to prepare fresh foods for infants and children. In the absence of refrigerators, foods prepared in advance have posed a major health threat to infants and children. Women's associations can help mothers to find a solution. In Peru, mothers' clubs have been formed to assist working mothers in safe infant feeding.

Insurance companies

Insurance companies should have a vested interest in the prevention of foodborne diseases as these are among the most widespread health problems and the cost in terms of claims and absenteeism from work may be considerable.

Insurance companies could collaborate with governments in disseminating information to travellers, the elderly and other vulnerable groups in order to minimize their health problems, and at the same time reduce the costs to the companies. In this context, the valuable collaboration of the British Life Assurance Trust with WHO in the preparation of an international list of audiovisual educational materials is an example of efforts made by an insurance organization in education in food safety.

Religious and other organizations with a humanitarian role

In some societies, religious groups have regulated the selection, preparation and consumption of food by their followers, in many instances because of safety concerns. Practically all religions encourage personal hygiene (*139*). Because of the influence that religious and social institutions have in communities, their involvement in food safety education can be of great value. In addition, in times of war, disaster or displacement, religious institutions and other humanitarian organizations are often involved in the preparation and distribution of food to the people affected. These groups can play a vital role in communicating the need for food safety and hygiene.

References

1. Motarjemi Y et al. Contaminated weaning food: a major risk factor for diarrhoea and associated malnutrition. *Bulletin of the World Health Organization*, 1993, 71(1):79–92.

2. Motarjemi Y et al. Contaminated food: a hazard for the very young. *World health forum*, 1994, 15(1):69–71.

3. Abdussalam M, Käferstein FK. Food safety in primary health care, *World health forum*, 1994, 15(4):393–399.

4. *Preventing foodborne illness: listeriosis.* Atlanta, GA, Centers for Disease Control and Prevention, 1992.

5. *Listeria infection and pregnancy.* Wellington, New Zealand Department of Health [brochure].

6. *While you are pregnant: safe eating and how to avoid infection from food and animals.* London, Department of Health [brochure].

7. *Listeriosis infection and pregnancy.* Perth, Department of Health of Western Australia, 1995.

8. *For pregnant women: dietary advice on listeriosis.* Canberra, National Food Authority of Australia [brochure].

9. *Mat för tvaa. Goda rad för dig som väntar barn. [Food for two. Good advice for you who are expecting a child.]* Uppsala, Livsmedelsverket, 1995 [poster].

10. *Maman, prends soin de toi et de moi. [Mama, take care of yourself and of me.]* Paris, Ministry of Social Affairs and Health, 1995 [brochure].

11. Newton LH, Hall SM. A survey of health education material for the primary prevention of congenital toxoplasmosis. *Communicable disease report*, 1995, 5(2):R21–R26.

12. *Protecting, promoting and supporting breast-feeding: the special role of maternity services. A joint WHO/UNICEF statement.* Geneva, World Health Organization, 1989.

13. *Breast-feeding. The technical basis and recommendations for action.* Geneva, World Health Organization, 1993 (unpublished document WHO/NUT/MCH/93.1; available on request from Nutrition, World Health Organization, 1211 Geneva 27, Switzerland).

14. Akré J. Infant feeding: the physiological basis. *Bulletin of the World Health Organization,* 1989, 67(supplement).

15. Amin-Zaki L et al. Perinatal methylmercury poisoning in Iraq. *American journal of diseases in children,* 1976, 130:1070–1076.

16. Blythe DG et al. Mother's milk turns toxic following fish feast. *Journal of the American Medical Association,* 1990, 264(16):2074.

17. Schutz D, Moy GG, Käferstein FK. *GEMS/Food International Dietary Survey: infant exposure to certain organochlorine contaminants from breast milk—a risk assessment.* Geneva, World Health Organization, 1998 (unpublished document WHO/FSF/FOS/98.4; available on request from Food Safety, World Health Organization, 1211 Geneva 27, Switzerland).

18. *Goda råd om fisk. [Good advice about fish.]* Uppsala, Livsmedelsverket, 1992.

19. Slorach S. Kvicksilver och andra främmande ämnen in fisk—aatgärder för att begränss hälsorkerna. [Measures to reduce health risk from mercury and other chemical contaminants in fish.] *Vaar Föda,* 1992, 44(2):163–170.

20. *PCBs, PCDDs and PCDFs in breast milk: assessment of health risks.* Copenhagen, World Health Organization Regional Office for Europe, 1988 (Environmental Health Series, No. 29).

21. Gobas F. *Selected persistent contaminants in human breast milk in the Great Lakes Basin.* Windsor, Ontario, The Great Lakes Institute, 1990.

22. HIV and infant feeding: an interim statement. *Weekly epidemiological record*, 1996, 71:289–296.

23. Bern C et al. The magnitude of the global problem of diarrhoeal disease: a ten-year update. *Bulletin of the World Health Organization*, 1992, 70(6):705–714.

24. Black RE et al. Contamination of weaning foods and transmission of enterotoxigenic *Escherichia coli* diarrhoea in children in rural Bangladesh. *Transactions of the Royal Society of Tropical Medicine and Hygiene*, 1982, 76(2):259–264.

25. Black RE et al. Enterotoxigenic *Escherichia coli* diarrhoea: acquired immunity and transmission in an endemic area. *Bulletin of the World Health Organization*, 1981, 59(2):263–268.

26. Henry FJ et al. Bacterial contamination of weaning foods and drinking water in rural Bangladesh. *Epidemiology and infection*, 1990, 104:79–85.

27. Barrel RAE, Rowland MGM. Infant foods as a potential source of diarrhoeal illness in rural West Africa. *Transactions of the Royal Society of Tropical Medicine and Hygiene*, 1979, 73(1):85–89.

28. Khin Nwe OO et al. Bacteriologic studies of food and water consumed by children in Myanmar: 1. The nature of contamination. *Journal of diarrhoeal disease research*, 1991, 9(2):87–90.

29. Black RE et al. Incidence and etiology of infantile diarrhea and major routes of transmission in Huascar, Peru. *American journal of epidemiology*, 1989, 129:785–799.

30. Michanie S et al. Critical control points for foods prepared in households in which babies had salmonellosis. *International journal of food microbiology*, 1987, 5:337–354.

31. Michanie S et al. Critical control points for foods prepared in households whose members had either alleged typhoid fever or diarrhea. *International journal of food microbiology*, 1988, 7:123–124.

32. Caparelli E, Mata LJ. Microflora of maize prepared as tortillas. *Applied microbiology*, 1975, 29:802–806.

33. Soundy J, Rivera H. Acute diarrhoeal diseases: longitudinal study in a sample of Salvadorean population II: Analysis of the faeces and foods. *Revista del Instituto de Investigaciones Médicas*, 1972, 1:307–316.

34. St Louis M et al. Epidemic cholera in West Africa: the role of food handling and high risk foods. *American journal of epidemiology*, 1990, 131(4):719–728.

35. *Report on street-vended and weaning foods in Yangon, Myanmar.* Geneva, World Health Organization, 1995 (unpublished document; available on request from Food Safety, World Health Organization, 1211 Geneva 27, Switzerland).

36. *Basic principles for the safe preparation of safe food for infants and young children.* Geneva, World Health Organization, 1996 (unpublished document WHO/FNU/FOS/96.6; available on request from Food Safety, World Health Organization, 1211 Geneva 27, Switzerland).

37. ICD/GTZ/SEAMO/WHO. *Food safety for nutritionists: a modular course on food safety.* Geneva, World Health Organization (in preparation).

38. *Training health workers in food safety*, Vol. 1 *Basic food safety for health workers.* Geneva, World Health Organization, 1998 (unpublished document; available on request from Food Safety, World Health Organization, 1211 Geneva 27, Switzerland) (Vol 2 in preparation).

39. *Teaching for better learning.* Geneva, World Health Organization, 1992.

40. *Education for health. A manual on health education in primary health care.* Geneva, World Health Organization, 1988.

41. *International travel and health: vaccination requirements and health advice.* Geneva, World Health Organization, 2000.

42. *A guide on safe food for travellers.* Geneva, World Health Organization, 1994 [brochure].

43. *Cholera: basic facts for travellers.* Geneva, World Health Organization [brochure].

44. *Get hooked on: important health information for people with immune disorders.* Washington, DC, Food and Drug Administration [brochure FDA 92-2261].

45. *Get hooked on: important health information for people with diabetes mellitus.* Washington, DC, Food and Drug Administration [brochure FDA 92-2258].

46. *Get hooked on: important health information for people with liver disease.* Washington, DC, Food and Drug Administration [brochure FDA 92-2260].

47. *WHO surveillance programme for control of foodborne infections and intoxications in Europe, fifth report (1985–1989), sixth report (1990–1992).* Berlin, Federal Institute for Health Protection of Consumers and Veterinary Medicine, 1992 and 1995.

48. Pollock AM, Whitty PM. Crisis in our hospital kitchen: ancillary staffing levels during an outbreak of food poisoning in a long-stay hospital. *British medical journal*, 1990, 300(6721):383–385.

49. Biering G et al. Three cases of neonatal meningitis caused by *Enterobacer sakazakii* in powdered milk. *Journal of clinical microbiology*, 1989, 27(9):2054–2056.

50. *Country report of Côte d'Ivoire to the FAO/WHO International Conference on Nutrition, Rome, 1992.* Rome, Food and Agriculture Organization of the United Nations, 1992.

51. Wood RC, MacDonald K, Osterholm MT. Campylobacter enteritis outbreaks associated with drinking raw milk during youth activities—a 10-year review of outbreaks in the United States. *Journal of the American Medical Association*, 1992, 268(22):3228–3230.

52. Guzman P. The role of teachers and homemakers in communicating food safety information and combatting misinformation. In: *Proceedings of the Second Asian Conference on Food Safety, Bangkok, Thailand, 18–23 September 1994.* Bangkok, International Life Sciences Institute, 1995.

53. Morely D. The very young as agents of change. *World health forum,* 1993, 14(1):23–24.

54. *Health promotion and community action for health in developing countries.* Geneva, World Health Organization, 1994.

55. *Facts for life. Lessons from experience.* New York, UNICEF, 1996.

56. Williams T, Moon A, Williams M. *Food, environment and health: a guide for primary school teachers.* Geneva, World Health Organization, 1990.

57. *Teacher's resource book: prototype action-oriented school health curriculum.* Alexandria, World Health Organization Regional Office for the Eastern Mediterranean, 1990.

58. *Comprehensive school health education: suggested guidelines for action.* Geneva, World Health Organization, 1992 (unpublished document WHO/UNESCO/UNICEF/92.2; available on request from Department of Health Promotion, World Health Organization, 1211 Geneva 27, Switzerland).

59. Arnhold W et al. *Healthy eating for young people in Europe: nutrition education in health promoting schools* (draft). Kiel, Ministry of Education of Schleswig-Holstein, 1995.

60. *Food hygiene with Hy-Genie.* London, Ministry of Agriculture, Fisheries and Food, 1994.

61. Ridgwell J. *Working with food in primary schools. A teacher's resource focusing on food hygiene and safety.* London, Ridgwell Press, 1996.

62. *Food safety resource.* Wellington, New Zealand Ministry of Health, 1993.

63. *Food safety: examples of health education materials.* Geneva, World Health Organization, 1989 (unpublished document WHO/EHE/FOS/89.2; available on request from Food Safety, World Health Organization, 1211 Geneva 27, Switzerland).

64. *Pied Crow's environment special magazine.* Nairobi, Care-Kenya (Health issue 4).

65. *Haamro Sathi (Our friend).* Kathmandu, Health Learning Materials Centre, 1993.

66. Scherer C. Strategies for communicating risks to the public. *Food technology,* 1991 (October):110–116.

67. Mossel DAA, Drake DM. Processing food for safety and reassuring the consumer. *Food technology,* 1990 (December):63–67.

68. Lee K. Food neophobia, major causes and treatments. *Food technology,* 1989 (December):62–73.

69. *Operation risk.* East Lansing, MI, Michigan University (Extension Children, Youth and Family Programs).

70. *Food technologies and public health.* Geneva, World Health Organization, 1995 (unpublished document WHO/FNU/FOS/95.12; available on request from Food Safety, World Health Organization, 1211 Geneva 27, Switzerland).

71. *Control of foodborne trematode infections. Report of a WHO Study Group.* Geneva, World Health Organization, 1995 (WHO Technical Report Series, No. 849).

72. Mathias RG. The effects of inspection frequency and food handler education on restaurant inspection violations. *Canadian journal of public health*, 1995, 86(1):46–50.

73. *Health surveillance and management procedures for food handling personnel. Report of a WHO consultation.* Geneva, World Health Organization, 1989 (WHO Technical Report Series, No. 785).

74. Jacob M. *Safe food handling: a training guide for managers of food service establishments.* Geneva, World Health Organization, 1989.

75. *Hygiene in mass catering: important rules.* Geneva, World Health Organization, 1994 (unpublished document WHO/FNU/FOS/94.5; available on request from Food Safety, World Health Organization, 1211 Geneva 27, Switzerland).

76. Prevention of foodborne hepatitis A. *Weekly epidemiological record*, 1993, 68(5):25–26.

77. Food safety measures for eggs and foods containing eggs. *Weekly epidemiological record*, 1993, 68(22):157–158.

78. *Code of hygienic practice for precooked and cooked foods in mass catering.* In: *Codex Alimentarius*, Vol. 1B. Rome, Food and Agriculture Organization of the United Nations, 1995.

79. *Application of the Hazard Analysis Critical Control Point (HACCP) system for the improvement of food safety. WHO supported case studies on food prepared in homes, at street vending operations, and in cottage industries.* Geneva, World Health Organization, 1993 (unpublished document WHO/FNU/FOS/93.1; available on request from Food Safety, World Health Organization, 1211 Geneva 27, Switzerland).

80. Bryan FL. *Hazard Analysis Critical Control Point evaluations—a guide to identifying hazards and assessing risks associated with food preparation and storage.* Geneva, World Health Organization, 1992.

81. *Training aspects of the Hazard Analysis Critical Control Point system. Report of a WHO workshop on training in HACCP with the pariticipation of FAO.* Geneva, World Health Organization, 1996 (unpublished document WHO/FNU/FOS/96.3; available on request from Food Safety, World Health Organization, 1211 Geneva 27, Switzerland).

82. *Health and environment in emergencies and disasters. A practical guide.* Geneva, World Health Organization (in preparation).

83. Clarke D. *An international directory of audiovisual material.* Geneva, World Health Organization, 1995 (unpublished document WHO/FNU/FOS/95.4; available on request from Food Safety, World Health Organization, 1211 Geneva 27, Switzerland).

84. Jacob M. Expo health controls. *International food safety news*, 1992, 1(8):65.

85. *The first certificate in food safety.* London, Royal Institute of Public Health and Hygiene, 1994.

86. *HACCP training standard: HACCP principles and their application in food safety.* London, Royal Institute of Public Health and Hygiene, 1995.

87. *Food hygiene microbiology courses.* Lymington, United Kingdom, The Society of Food Hygiene Technology.

88. *Food safe: foodhandler training programme.* Training package. Victoria Park, WA, Australian Institute of Environmental Health.

89. *Food hygiene training: a guide to its responsible management.* London, Institute of Food Science and Technology, 1992.

90. Jacob M. Salmonella in poultry—is there a solution? *Environmental policy and practice,* 1995, 5(2):75–80.

91. Council Directive 93/43/EEC on the hygiene of foodstuffs. *Official Journal of the European Communities,* 1993:L175/1–L175/11.

92. Taylor E. Is food hygiene training really effective? *Environmental health,* 1996:275–276.

93. Ehiri JE, Morris G. Hygiene training and education of food handlers: does it work? *Ecology of food and nutrition,* 1996, 35:243–251.

94. Smith RA. Thoughts on a national food hygiene training policy. *Health and hygiene,* 1994, 15:103–108.

95. *Guide on safe food for travellers.* Geneva, World Health Organization, 1994.

96. *Halsorad for utlands resenar. [Health messages for overseas travellers.]* Stockholm, Apoteksbolaget, 1992 [brochure].

97. *Proceedings of the WHO/WTO Regional Conference for Africa and the Mediterranean, Tunis, Tunisia, 25–27 November 1991.* Madrid, World Tourism Organization, 1992.

98. *Proceedings of Inter-American Conference on Food Protection and Tourism, Cancun, Mexico, 15–17 November 1992.* Washington, DC, Pan American Health Organization, 1993.

99. *Proceedings of the WHO/WTO Regional Conference for Africa and the Mediterranean, Tunis, Tunisia, 26–28 November 1998.* Madrid, World Tourism Organization, 1999.

100. *Essential safety requirements for street-vended foods.* Geneva, World Health Organization, 1996 (unpublished document WHO/FNU/FOS/96.7; available on request from Food Safety, World Health Organization, 1211 Geneva 27, Switzerland).

101. *Street foods.* Rome, Food and Agriculture Organization of the United Nations, 1997 (FAO Food and Nutrition Paper, No. 63).

102. Oltersdorf U. Differences in German consumer concerns over suggested health and food hazards. In: Feichtinger E, Köhler BM, eds. *Current research into eating practices. Contribution of social sciences. 16th Annual Scientific Meeting of AGEV, Potsdam, Germany, 14–16 October 1993.* Supplement to *Ernährungs-Umschau [Nutrition survey],* 1995, 42:171–173.

103. Mortimore SE. *How effective are the current sources of food hygiene education and training in shaping behaviour?* [Thesis] Leicester, University of Leicester Centre for Labour Market Studies, 1993.

104. Griffith CL, Mathias KA, Price PE. The mass media and food hygiene education. *British food journal,* 1994, 96(9):16–21.

105. *Lebensmittel-vergiftungen: wie man sich schutzt. [Food poisoning: how to protect oneself.]* Vienna, Ministry for Health, Sport and Consumer Protection, 1993.

106. *Wie vermeidet man Lebensmittel-vergiftungen? [How does one avoid food poisoning?]* Cologne, Federal Office for Health Promotion, 1985.

107. *Preventing foodborne illness: a guide to safe food handling.* Washington, DC, United States Department of Agriculture, 1990.

108. *If you eat raw oysters, you need to know.* Washington, DC, Food and Drug Administration (brochure FDA 95-2293).

109. *Food for thought: a handbook on food safety and hygiene.* Singapore, Ministry of the Environment, 1989.

110. *Assure safe catering: a management system for hazard analysis.* London, Department of Health, 1993.

111. *Food poisoning: what you need to know.* Perth, Health Department of Western Australia, 1995 [brochure].

112. *Basic food is best.* Pretoria, Consumer Council [brochure].

113. *Food safety: a guide to safe food handling.* Perth, Health Department of Western Australia, 1994 [brochure].

114. *The shoppers's guide to food safety.* Perth, Health Department of Western Australia, 1993 [brochure].

115. *Hats and food handlers.* Perth, Health Department of Western Australia, 1994 [brochure].

116. *Campylobacter gastroenteritis.* Perth, Health Department of Western Australia, 1993 [brochure].

117. *How safe are food additives?* Perth, Health Department of Western Australia, 1990 [brochure].

118. *How safe is lead crystal?* Perth, Health Department of Western Australia, 1992 [brochure].

119. *Cleaning and sanitising.* Perth, Health Department of Western Australia, 1995 [brochure].

120. *Simple rules for safe sandwiches.* Perth, Health Department of Western Australia, 1993 [brochure].

121. *Amoebiasis.* Melbourne, Department of Health and Community Services of Victoria, 1995 [brochure].

122. *Cryptosporidium.* Melbourne, Department of Health and Community Services of Victoria, 1995 [brochure].

123. *Hepatitis A.* Melbourne, Department of Health and Community Services of Victoria, 1995 [brochure].

124. *Listeriosis.* Melbourne, Department of Health and Community Services of Victoria, 1995 [brochure].

125. *Food poisoning and how to prevent it.* Melbourne, Department of Health and Community Services of Victoria, 1995 [brochure].

126. *Safe food storage and displaying.* Melbourne, Department of Health and Community Services of Victoria, 1995 [brochure].

127. *Salmonellosis.* Melbourne, Department of Health and Community Services of Victoria, 1995.

128. *Hygienic food preparation and handling.* Melbourne, Department of Health and Community Services of Victoria, 1995.

129. *Personal hygiene for people working with food.* Melbourne, Department of Health and Community Services of Victoria, 1995.

130. *For asthma sufferers. The facts about sulphites in food.* Canberra, Australian National Food Authority.

131. *Food fact file.* London, BBC Education, 1992.

132. Allen RJL, Käferstein FK. Foodborne disease, food hygiene and consumer education. *Archiv für Lebensmittelhygiene (Archive for food hygiene)*, 1983, 34(4):86–89.

133. *Primary health care. Report of the International Conference of Primary Health Care, Alma-Ata, 6–12 September 1978.* Geneva, World Health Organization, 1978 ("Health for All" Series, No. 1).

134. *Report of food safety labelling.* Toronto, Ontario Ministry of Agriculture, Food and Rural Affairs, 1996.

135. Young M. Light on food safety. *World health forum*, 1992, 12(4):400–402.

136. *Foodborne illness: its origin and how to avoid it.* Brussels, European Food Information Council, 1996.

137. *Children's view on food and nutrition. A pan-European survey.* Brussels, European Food Information Council, 1995.

138. Hospedales J et al. Private sector response against the cholera threat in Trinidad and Tobago. *Bulletin of the Pan American Health Organization*, 1993, 27(4):331–336.

139. Health education in food safety. Report of a WHO consultation. Geneva, World Health Organization, 1988 (unpublished document WHO/EHE/FOS/88.7; available on request from Food Safety, World Health Organization, 1211 Geneva 27, Switzerland).

140. Abdussalam M. Islamic rules governing food. *Hamdard*, 1989, 32(4):17–26.

CHAPTER 5

Implementation of health education in food safety

Problems, sociocultural features and resources vary from country to country. It is therefore not possible to devise a plan of action or provide a curriculum for a food safety education programme which would be globally applicable. Each country or area considering a food safety education programme or intervention should develop a programme and plan of action that are relevant to its needs, population characteristics and infrastructure. Programme and intervention are considered as alternatives. This chapter applies both to broad national programmes for the education of consumers and food handlers, as well as to specific educational activities.

There are many valuable publications on the implementation of health education programmes (*1–3*). This chapter aims to recommend the key elements of a plan for health education in food safety (Fig. 12), provide guidance on issues of food safety, and draw on some experiences in this area. The key elements recommended in this chapter can be applied in a national programme, as well as in training and educational activities targeted at specific groups such as small communities or the staff of food service establishments.

Recognition, commitment and resources

Political recognition and endorsement of the aims and objectives of a food safety education programme, and support from prominent community leaders and institutions concerned with food safety, are essential to the success of such a programme.

Thus, the first step towards health education in food safety is to raise the awareness of policy-makers on the importance of foodborne diseases and the role of health education in food safety, ascertaining their commitment to integrating education in food safety into national food and nutrition policies and related public health policies. Resources for the implementation of the programme also need to be identified or made available. The confidence and enthusiasm of policy-makers and the general community regarding the programme should be stimulated so that everyone has a sense of involvement and commitment to its success. Box 25 shows some of the commitments made at international level by policy-makers in support of food safety and health education programmes. These policy statements may be used by managers of food safety and health education programmes to obtain support for health education in food safety.

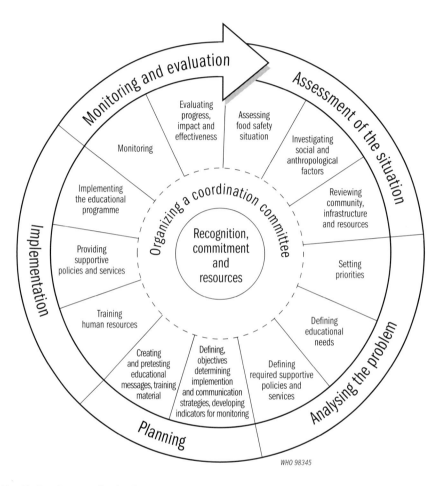

WHO 98345

Fig. 12. Key elements of a plan for health education in food safety

---

Box 25. International policy statements supporting health education in food safety

■ One of the fundamental principles of primary health care is the participation of the community at all stages. For communities to be intelligently involved, they need to have easy access to the right kind of information concerning their health situation and how they themselves can help to improve it.

■ ... primary health care should include at least education concerning prevailing health problems and the methods of identifying, preventing and controlling them ...

■ . . . as part of total coverage of populations through primary health care, high priority be given to the special needs of women, children, working populations at high risk, and the underprivileged segments of society, and that the necessary activities be maintained, reaching out into all homes and working places to identify systematically those at highest risk, to provide continuing care to them, and to eliminate factors contributing to ill health.

WHO/UNICEF International Conference on Primary Health Care, Alma-Ata, 1978

■ Consumer education and information programmes should cover such important aspects of consumer protection as the following: [a] health, nutrition, prevention of food-borne diseases and food adulteration.

United Nations Guidelines for Consumer Protection, 1986

■ Where appropriate, governments, in close cooperation with interested parties, should . . . support consumer education to contribute to an educated and knowledgeable public, safe practices in the home, community participation and active consumer associations.

FAO/WHO International Conference on Nutrition, Rome, 1992

■ . . . empowerment of people and community participation were seen as essential factors in a democratic health promotion approach and the driving force for self-reliance and development . . . education is a basic human right and a key element in bringing about the political, economic and social changes needed to make health a possibility for all. Education should be accessible throughout life and be built on the principle of equity, particularly with respect to culture, social class and gender.

International Conference on Health Promotion, Sundsvall, 1991

■ The Forty-sixth World Health Assembly . . . urges Member States . . . to contain and reduce the rate at which the prevalence of diet-related diseases and of conditions related to them is rising.

World Health Assembly Resolution 46.7 (1993)

■ The Forty-second World Health Assembly . . . urgently calls upon Member States . . . to develop, in the spirit of the Alma-Ata, Ottawa and Adelaide conferences, strategies for health promotion and health education as an essential element of primary health care, and to strengthen the required infrastructure and resources at all levels.

World Health Assembly Resolution 42.44 (1989)

Coordination

Education in food safety has a greater chance of success if all concerned sectors are appropriately involved. While the public health sector has to play the leading and coordinating role, it must take steps to involve representatives of other sectors, both governmental (e.g. education, agriculture, tourism, local government) and nongovernmental (e.g. industry, universities and research institutes, consumer groups), through an interdisciplinary committee or similar mechanism (*4, 5*).

The organizing committee will be responsible for the management of the programme. Its tasks could include:

— assessing the situation;
— determining the problems, setting priorities and defining specific needs with regard to food safety education;
— developing a plan, including defining objectives and policies, identifying strategies for implementation of the programme, and determining its time frame;
— determining the responsibilities of each sector in the implementation process;
— mobilizing resources;
— securing supportive policies and services, including qualified and trained human resources, regulations as appropriate and other health services;
— monitoring progress and evaluating the impact of interventions;
— making changes in the ongoing activities as necessary, and planning future activities.

In many countries it may also be appropriate to develop a decentralized system and to establish a national committee as well as regional and/or local committees. In this case, the functions of the national committee could be to provide guidance and policy, support training of human resources, and coordinate activities at national level, while the regional or local committees would assess the situation in their regions, set priorities, adapt national policies, implement the programme, monitor progress and evaluate it.

Assessment of the situation

Health education in food safety should be culture-specific. It must also respond to the health, technological, social and economic situations that prevail in a particular society or in particular cultural or social groups. The educational programme or intervention should take into account problems and needs that are specific to the target groups. It should therefore be based on a combination of two types of information: technical information on food safety problems and practices that lead to foodborne illness, and underlying sociocultural and economic factors that influence food safety. The educational programme should also take into account the resources available and the characteristics of the target population. The latter will influence the strategies for implementing the programme. Where such data are not available, research studies may need to be initiated prior to planning and implementing the programme. Universities and other research and educational institutes can facilitate this kind of study. The assessment of the situation and the identification of problems would benefit from being carried out by a multidisciplinary team that includes epidemiologists, food scientists[1] and anthropologists.

Food safety situation

Various types of information may be needed. The assessment of the food safety situation should include collection of technical data on foodborne diseases, food contamination, dietary habits and food preparation practices.

Epidemiological surveillance data on foodborne diseases and/or monitoring data on food contamination

Statistics on foodborne diseases, including morbidity and mortality, are needed to assess the nature and magnitude of the diseases and their health and economic implications. Such data are important for prioritizing foodborne diseases and determining the measures that are needed. Epidemiological data on foodborne disease outbreaks also increase understanding of risk factors that lead to foodborne diseases and help in identifying high-risk foods, operations and practices. Such data may be obtained through foodborne disease surveillance programmes, where these exist.

The data collected through food contamination monitoring programmes can be used to assess whether the foods in question may present health risks for the population or for subgroups. Such programmes are particularly important for preventing or limiting the exposure of populations to chemical contaminants.

Foodborne hazards and control measures

Scientific information on foodborne hazards includes the ecology of microorganisms, the toxicological effects of chemicals, and possible control measures for preventing contamination, reducing or eliminating hazards or controlling growth and production of toxins. Such data will improve

---

[1] The term is used in a broad sense to mean food scientists and technologists, food engineers, food microbiologists, veterinary surgeons, toxicologists, chemists, food inspectors, and other scientists with expertise in food.

understanding of potential health risks and the possible consequences of food preparation practices.

Data on food preparation practices based on HACCP studies

HACCP studies will increase understanding of the behaviour or food preparation practices which are critical for food safety and which should be modified or reinforced. These studies should be carried out on foods or food preparation procedures that have been identified as high risk by foodborne disease surveillance and/or food contamination monitoring programmes. They can be regarded as complementary to epidemiological investigation of foodborne diseases with respect to identifying risk factors and behaviour which need to be modified or reinforced. They can also be used to identify problems where surveillance programmes do not exist or are weak.

Food pattern

The type of food eaten, and its source, should also be assessed. The types of information that may be useful in the assessment are: agricultural practices and food processing (if, for instance, there is the possibility that a raw foodstuff reaches the market contaminated), foods imported (the type of high-risk foods that are imported, and whether the food control infrastructure is effectiv enough to prevent contaminated foodstuffs from reaching the local market), environmental hazards (e.g. whether a safe water supply is available, whether environmental contaminants may jeopardize the safety of the food), and how they affect raw foodstuffs, food consumption and preparation habits (e.g whether preparation is adequate to prevent and control hazards, whether people have a predilection for certain high-risk foods, and food habits during travel).

Other types of information

Other types of information such as experiences and observations of food and health inspectors, health care workers, food producers and food service establishments should also be taken into account.

Factors underlying food-related behaviour

Social and anthropological information on food-related behaviour is needed to get to know the target population and understand the factors that underlie food preferences or food preparation practices. Information could be collected on the following (see page 81):

— predisposing factors (e.g. knowledge, attitudes, skills, beliefs and perceptions of the target population with regard to food safety, foodborne hazards and control measures);

— enabling factors (e.g. environmental conditions, economic situation, regulations and services such as water supply, sanitation and food storage facilities);

— reinforcing factors (e.g. whether the environment encourages safe habits or safe food handling through such measures as the certification of trained food handlers, the attitudes of managers or supervisors in food service establishments, and the requirements of consumers).

Community, infrastructure and resources

For the purposes of planning and implementation, it is also necessary to obtain demographic information on the community and data on its infrastructure and resources.

Demographic data

These include data on the population of the community and its age distribution (e.g. number of children, elderly), the number of households, the number of other vulnerable individuals (e.g. those infected with HIV), the number of travellers and their destination, numbers of immigrants and ethnic groups and their religion, the level of education and the proportion of illiterate persons, socioeconomic status and access to media, schools and health centres, and the proportion of the population living in urban or rural areas.

Food businesses

These data include information on the number and type of food industries, food and catering establishments, retailers and street food vendors.

Social institutions and resources

Here is included information on institutions that have an advocacy role and could be used to implement the educational programme. Examples are churches of various denominations, temples, mosques, schools, markets and other gathering places, health centres, travel agencies and so on.

System of communication

An inventory could be made of formal means of communication, such as newspapers, journals, radio stations, television channels, libraries and poster sites.

Analysis of problems

The results of the assessment should lead to the analysis and identification of problems, and to setting priorities, selecting appropriate strategies, defining educational needs and providing supportive policies and services.

Planning and implementation

Following identification of problems and educational needs, a plan should be developed. The plan should specify priorities, define objectives and determine strategies for communication and for the training and education of various target groups or population groups (Table 13). The plan should also determine the need for qualified and trained human resources, supportive policies and other services as well as the means to achieve them. The selection of strategies and partners for implementation should take into consideration the characteristics of the population and the existing infrastructure.

As part of the planning and implementation process, training material and

Table 13. Partners in education in food safety by target population

Partners for implementation	Target population
Public health services (primary health care centres, clinics, hospitals, physicians)	Mothers of small children High-risk groups (elderly, children, immunocompromised individuals, pregnant women, travellers), general public
Maternal and child health centres	Pregnant women, lactating women, mothers of infants and young children
Academia (universities, research institutes)	Health workers, public health professionals, food scientists, food inspectors, policy-makers
Secondary and primary schools	Children and adolescents, teachers, parents
Professional schools	Professional food handlers (cooks, waiters/waitresses), managers of hotels and restaurants
Food industry, including food service and catering establishments	Professional food handlers, consumers, supermarkets and retailers
Supermarkets and retailers	Professional and domestic food handlers
Mass media	Policy-makers and the general public
Food inspectors (consumer affairs bureau)	Consumers, food industry, food service and catering establishments, street food vendors
Consumer groups	Consumers and policy-makers
Religious and social institutions	Consumers (particularly socially disadvantaged)
Tourism sector (travel agencies, tour operators)	Travellers, food service and catering establishments
Local police	Street food vendors, retailers, food service establishments

educational messages need to be developed for the different target groups. This involves translating the technical and scientific information into training programmes and educational messages that are readily understood and accepted by the target population, taking into account their culture and socioeconomic situation. In this context, the expertise of communication and health education specialists is essential.

Before launching a long-term programme it may be necessary to carry out a pilot study to test its efficacy. Pretesting of educational material is also important to ensure that the message is understood correctly. The training material and educational messages can be tested for clarity and accuracy on a small group representative of the general audience. Pretesting of educational material is particularly important when it is used with persons of different cultures.

At the planning and implementation stages it is also important to consider indicators which will be used in monitoring and evaluation. This will enable constraints to be identified and remedial actions taken if necessary.

Monitoring and evaluation

Even when an educational programme is well designed and implemented, monitoring and evaluation can significantly contribute to its improvement. They should be considered as integral parts of each programme; they should take place as the programme proceeds and when it ends (6).

The purpose of evaluation is to ascertain whether the intervention has been successful. Evaluation also helps to identify changes that may be desirable or necessary in the programme. Pretesting of educational materials and the research studies mentioned above are themselves forms of evaluation.

Depending on the results of the evaluation it may be necessary to change the plan. The plan, including the objectives and priorities, may also need to be revised as a result of changes in the epidemiology of foodborne diseases, levels of food contaminants, food production systems, emerging pathogens or technologies, lifestyles (including international travel and migration), and natural or manmade environmental disasters and emergencies.

Evaluation can be carried out with regard to the criteria listed in Table 13. Evaluation may sometimes require additional HACCP studies, social and anthropological studies, or analysis of foodborne disease surveillance and food contamination monitoring data.

Lessons learned from health education

Many health education initiatives have failed because initial assumptions were only partially valid, or were not valid at all.

Table 13. Criteria for evaluation of food safety education programmes (Source: 6)

Criterion	Definition	Examples of application
Effectiveness	The degree of attainment of predetermined objectives.	Have food handlers' practices improved, resulting in a lower risk of food contamination? Has the level of knowledge increased, and behaviour changed? What percentage of food handlers has adopted the desired behaviour?
Impact	The overall effect on health and related socioeconomic development.	What is the overall effect on health and related socioeconomic development? Has there been a decrease in foodborne diseases or related economic costs?
Efficiency	The relationship between the results obtained and the resources expended.	What is the relationship between the results obtained (decrease in incidence of foodborne diseases or number of food handlers trained) and resources spent?
Progress	The comparison of actual with scheduled activities to ensure that operations are proceeding as planned and as scheduled.	Did the programme go as planned? How many food handlers have been trained compared with the number originally planned? How many households have been covered compared with the planned number?
Adequacy	Whether sufficient attention has been paid to certain previously determined courses of action.	Has the programme adequately covered all the target audiences? Has sufficient attention been paid to vulnerable groups (e.g. infants, the elderly, pregnant women)?
Relevance	The rationale for selecting behaviour in terms of its relevance to foodborne diseases as well as the social and economic consequences.	Is the behaviour being changed relevant to the foodborne diseases in question (e.g. hand-washing will not be relevant to prevention of botulism)?

Need for supportive policies and services

Education can be effective when conditions permit implementation of the recommendations and advice. For instance, tremendous efforts are being made by international organizations such as WHO and UNICEF, as well as by national authorities, to promote breastfeeding. Despite these efforts and the resources invested, in many countries women working outside the home find it difficult to breastfeed their babies (7). Lack of time may sometimes also lead to unsafe food preparation practices and in some poor populations causes contamination of complementary foods. As long as a national policy on maternity leave does not provide a solution for mothers in employment, there is little chance that education will bring about a change in behaviour.

Similarly, when water is not available, or there are no facilities for cold storage, or fuel is expensive or difficult to obtain, it may be difficult for poor households or urban dwellers to observe food safety principles, no matter how much education or training is given.

It is essential that the intervention or message is adapted to the conditions of the target population. For example, when refrigerators are not available, people can be advised not to store leftovers at room temperature for an extended time but to prepare food for one meal at a time. There is, of course, a limit to the extent to which education can be adapted to local conditions. If water is unsafe and households cannot afford, or do not have access to, fuel to boil their drinking-water or cook/reheat their food properly, there can be no assurance of food safety. Education in food safety under these conditions cannot bring about change.

It must be clearly borne in mind that health education cannot replace essential services. Policy-makers should therefore ensure that supporting policies and services are in place. Policy-makers should also take into consideration the implications of all policies that may directly or indirectly affect food safety. For example, in one country it has been observed that when the tax for imported fertilizers increased, farmers used sewage water to irrigate and fertilize their crops. This resulted in an epidemic of cholera due to contamination of vegetables. Similarly, an increase in the cost of fuel may negatively influence food preparation practices in poor social settings.

For health education in food safety to have any chance of success, it is imperative that measures to improve related policies and services are integrated into the overall food safety programme. A study in several countries in the Americas illustrated the importance of a supportive environment in the successful implementation of health education in food safety. Appreciation of the importance of hygienic handling by consumers and their demand for safe food constitute important reinforcing factors in the training and education of food handlers (Box 26).

Knowledge alone is very important but sometimes not sufficient

Health education is often based on the sole assumption that knowledge leads to the correct attitude, which then results in safe and healthy practices thereafter. This is unfortunately a false assumption. Food safety education programmes in industrialized countries have for years provided knowledge on simple hygiene procedures, such as the need to wash one's hands after using the toilet, that prevent food contamination. However, observation of actual food-handling practices, and reports of epidemiological investigations following incidents of foodborne disease, continue to show that deficient habits persist among food

---

Box 26. Trained street food vendors revert to old habits (8)

During 1995 and 1996, the Pan American Health Organization conducted a study to evaluate microbial contamination of street foods sold in eight Latin American cities.

In all, 2433 samples were analysed for the presence of *Vibrio cholerae*, *Staphylococcus aureus*, *Bacillus cereus* and *Clostridium perfringens* in doses sufficiently high to promote the appearance of clinical symptoms in consumers. The samples were also tested for the presence of *Salmonella* and *Escherichia coli* O157 : H7. The samples were collected from the most consumed food items in each city, with special attention to ready-to-eat preparations.

It was observed that the following microorganisms were present in doses infective to the consumers: *S. aureus* (8.42%); *B. cereus* (7.89%); *C. perfringens* (5.07%). *Salmonella* was present in 0.95% of the samples and *E. coli* O157 : H7 was found in one sample. This was the first documented finding of that emergent pathogen in street foods.

It was also found that much of the effort made in training street food handlers did not produce significant changes in the contamination of the food prepared by them. Most of the hygienic procedures taught to food handlers, like wearing special or clean clothes, washing hands frequently, and using disposable utensils, create additional costs that ultimately must be passed on to consumers. Since the consumers are not usually informed of the benefits of buying from trained vendors, and cannot easily identify them, they tend to select food by price. As a consequence, the trained food vendors soon returned to their previous practices.

---

handlers. The problem is more general than food safety. About 150 years have passed since the discovery by Ignaz Semmelweis of the importance of hand-washing in the control of infections in women during delivery. However, even today many physicians, in both developing and industrialized countries, neglect to wash their hands before examining each patient (*9, 10*). To bring about a change in behaviour, therefore, it is important to understand the reasons behind behaviour and the sociocultural factors that influence them. This points to the importance of social and anthropological research and integration of the findings into the educational programme or intervention.

It is important to remember that health education should not be based only on the provision of knowledge, but should aim "to foster activities that encourage people to *want* to be healthy, *know* how to stay healthy, *do* what they can individually and collectively to maintain health, and *seek* help when needed" (*11*).

The dichotomy between "real needs" and "felt needs"

People have a number of needs. Behaviours may depend on these needs, particularly if they are "felt" needs. In describing their needs, people determine a hierarchy—some needs are more important than others and some may be related to their own perception of risks. Quite often the needs people feel they have differ from their "real needs" based on health risks and as seen by the health authorities. The challenge for health workers and behavioural scientists is to create an educational atmosphere in which a real need (based on prevention of a health risk) becomes a felt need for the person or persons concerned.

Failures in the planning process

Health education should be based on the epidemiology of diseases and pathogens, on behaviours, and on the social and cultural factors that underlie those behaviours. The selection of behaviour to be modified should be based on scientific facts. Modifying it should have a significant impact on health. Many resources have been wasted promoting behaviour that has little or no relevance to the health problem. For example, for the prevention of diarrhoeal diseases, a number of projects have placed the main emphasis on protecting food from flies, and have linked the increase in the number of diarrhoeal disease cases during the summer to the increase in the number of flies. Others have investigated the presence of toys, baby bottles or dirty diapers without questioning the hygienic quality of the food prepared. The influence of poor hygienic handling of food on the incidence of diarrhoeal diseases has often been overlooked. Many studies have promoted hand hygiene without referring to its importance in connection with food preparation.

Many studies have also questioned the effectiveness of giving information and advice to travellers to try to prevent travel-related diseases. However, it should be admitted that in many instances the advice given to travellers is poor, incomplete, and sometimes not relevant to their destination.

While education and training in food safety are important for the prevention of foodborne diseases, it should be remembered that poor or erroneous education is likely to do more harm than good.

References

1. *Education for health: a manual for health education in primary health care.* Geneva, World Health Organization, 1992.

2. *The community health worker.* Geneva, World Health Organization, 1987.

3. Green LW, Kreuter M. *Health promotion planning: an educational and environmental approach.* Mountain View, CA, Mayfield Publishing Company, 1991.

4. *Food Safety Education Committee report: Proceedings of the Conference for Food Protection, San Jose, California, 12–16 March 1994.* Chicago, IL, Educational Foundation of the National Restaurant Association, 1994.

5. *Health promotion and community action for health in developing countries.* Geneva, World Health Organization, 1994.

6. *Evaluation of programmes to ensure food safety.* Geneva, World Health Organization, 1989.

7. *WHO global data bank on breast-feeding.* Geneva, World Health Organization, 1996 (unpublished document WHO/NUT/96.1; available on request from Nutrition for Health and Development, World Health Organization, 1211 Geneva 27, Switzerland).

8. Almeida C et al. *Contaminación microbiana de los alimentos vendidos en la via pública. [Microbial contamination of street foods.]* Washington, DC, Pan American Health Organization, 1996 (unpublished document OPS/HCP/HCV/FOS/96.22; available on request from Pan American Health Organization, 525, 23rd Street, NW, Washington, DC, 20037 USA).

9. Meengs MR et al. Hand washing frequency in emergency departments. *Annals of emergency medicine*, 1994, 23:1307–1312.

10. Jarvis WR. Handwashing—the Semmelweis lesson forgotten? *Lancet*, 1994, 344:1311–1312.

11. *New approaches to health education in primary health. Report of a WHO Expert Committee.* Geneva, World Health Organization, 1983 (WHO Technical Report Series, No. 609).

CHAPTER 6
Conclusion

Foodborne diseases are a major health and economic problem in both industrialized and developing countries. Policy-makers should recognize that the nutritional well-being of the population depends as much on availability of and access to nutritious food as on food safety (Box 27). The prevention of foodborne diseases through health education in food safety is both possible and cost-effective.

In view of the size of the task, solving the food safety problem may not be easy, particularly in many developing countries with limited resources. However, it should be realized that education is a powerful and practical means of improving public health both substantially and sustainably. Education has a lasting effect in preventing foodborne diseases by stimulating individuals and communities to want safe food, to appreciate food hazards, to learn how to control them and to observe the principles of food safety. Education enables people to make informed choices.

> **Box 27. The importance of food safety for human nutrition (*FAO/WHO International Conference on Nutrition, 1992*)**
>
> The causes of nutritional problems are broad, and eliminating malnutrition and overnutrition is not merely a matter of increasing or altering food supplies. Rather, the causes of nutritional problems are likely to be complex, and interdependent, and clearly extend to food quality and safety.

The public health sector has a crucial role to play in food safety education. In cooperation with other governmental sectors (such as tourism, education, agriculture, municipalities) and nongovernmental sectors (such as industry, universities, research institutes, consumer groups, religious groups), the public health sector should develop and implement a programme for the education of food handlers and the general public. This could include:

— development and dissemination of educational materials for consumers;

— implementation of food safety education campaigns and programmes using mass media and other channels of communication;

— establishment of a consumer affairs bureau where consumers can obtain answers to their queries;

— integration of food safety into the primary health care programme, with specific emphasis on the education of mothers (or other persons looking after small children) and vulnerable groups;

— integration of food safety into the curricula of primary and secondary schools;
— integration of food safety into training curricula for health workers and nutritionists;
— integration of food safety into the curricula of hotel and restaurant schools;
— mandatory education and training of professional food handlers, particularly managers of food service establishments;
— dissemination of information on high-risk foods to travellers;
— training and education of street food vendors in the basic rules of food safety.

It is hoped that this book will make a positive contribution to the quest for increased health education in food safety.

Foodborne illnesses: some facts and figures

The following tables provide concise information about the epidemiology of foodborne diseases and how they can be prevented. The tables give the name (and alternative names) of foodborne illnesses, together with the following information about each of them:

— the codes by which the illness is classified in the International Classification of Diseases, 9th and 10th revisions (ICD-9 and ICD-10);
— the etiological agent that causes the illness;
— the main characteristics of the etiological agent;
— the incubation period of the illness;
— the symptoms;
— the possible sequelae of the illness;
— the duration of the illness;
— the reservoir or source of the etiological agent;
— the mode of transmission of the agent, together with examples of foods that have been involved in outbreaks;
— measures that can be taken to control/prevent the spread of the etiological agent (by industry, by professional and domestic food handlers, and by consumers);
— the occurrence of the illness, as indicated by + (less than 1 case per 100000 population), ++ (1–100 cases per 100000 population) and +++ (over 100 cases per 100000 population);
— the geographical occurrence of the illness;
— other details about the nature of the illness or about the agent that causes it.

The diseases are listed in alphabetical order by type of pathogen, with bacteria first, then viruses and then parasites (protozoa, nematodes, cestodes, trematodes).

Type of illness	*Aeromonas* enteritis
Etiological agent	Bacterium: *Aeromonas hydrophila*.
Characteristics of the agent	Gram-negative, motile, non-spore-forming, facultatively anaerobic, straight or curved rods that will not grow in 4–5% salt or at pH < 6. Optimum growth temperature is 28 °C, but growth may occur at lower temperatures, down to 4 °C. Many strains have the ability to grow over a wide pH range (4–10) under otherwise optimal conditions.
Incubation period	24–48 hours.
Symptoms	Watery stools, stomach cramps, mild fever and vomiting.
Sequelae	Bronchopneumonia, cholecystitis.
Duration	Days–weeks.
Reservoir/source	A common organism found in aquatic environments that has been isolated from a wide range of foods.
Mode of transmission and example of foods involved in outbreaks	Seafood (fish, shrimp, oysters), snails, drinking-water.
Specific control measures	*Industrial:* treatment and disinfection of water supplies, food irradiation. *Food service establishment/household:* thorough cooking of food, no long-term refrigeration of ready-to-eat foods.
Occurrence	Worldwide. Sporadic outbreaks have been reported from Africa, Australia, Europe, Japan and North America. Estimated rate of occurrence: unknown.
Other comments	Opportunistic pathogen.

Type of illness	***Bacillus cereus* gastroenteritis** a) Diarrhoeal syndrome b) Emetic syndrome
ICD code	ICD-9: 005.8 ICD-10: A05.4
Etiological agent	Bacterial toxin: a) Diarrhoeal syndrome due to production of heat-labile toxins either in the gut or in food. b) Emetic syndrome due to heat-stable toxins produced in food.
Characteristics of the agent	Gram-positive, facultatively anaerobic, motile rods which produce heat-resistant spores; generally mesophilic, growing between 10 °C and 50 °C, with the optimum at 28–37 °C (there are, however, psychrotrophic strains which grow at 4 °C). They will grow in a pH range of 4.3–9.3 and water activity (a_w) above 0.92. Spores are moderately heat-resistant, and survive freezing and drying. Some strains require heat activation for spores to germinate and outgrow.
Incubation period	a) Diarrhoeal syndrome: 8–16 hours. b) Emetic syndrome: 1–5 hours.
Symptoms	a) Diarrhoeal syndrome: acute diarrhoea, nausea and abdominal pain. b) Emetic syndrome: acute nausea, vomiting and abdominal pain and sometimes diarrhoea.
Duration	a) Diarrhoeal syndrome: 24–36 hours. b) Emetic syndrome: 24–36 hours.
Reservoir/source	Widely distributed in nature (soil).
Mode of transmission and example of foods involved in outbreaks	Ingestion of food that has been stored at ambient temperatures after cooking, permitting the growth of bacterial spores and production of toxin. Many outbreaks (particularly those of emetic syndrome) are associated with cooked or fried rice that has been kept at ambient temperature. Examples of foods involved include starchy products, such as boiled or fried rice, spices, dried foods, milk and dairy products, vegetable dishes and sauces.
Specific control measures	*Food service establishment/household:* Effective temperature control to prevent spore germination and growth: food storage at >60 °C or properly refrigerated at <10 °C until use, unless other factors such as pH or a_w are such as to prevent growth. When refrigeration facilities are not available, cook only quantities required for immediate consumption. Toxins associated with emetic syndrome are heat-resistant and reheating, including stir frying, will not destroy them.
Occurrence	Worldwide. Estimated rate of occurrence: ++/+++.

Type of illness	Botulism
ICD code	ICD-9: 005.1 ICD-10: A05.1
Etiological agent	Bacterial toxin: toxins of *Clostridium botulinum*.
Characteristics of the agent	Gram-positive, spore-forming, obligately anaerobic, motile rods which produce seven potent neurotoxins A–G; only A, B, E and, infrequently, F have been associated with disease (*Clostridium botulinum*). Group G is named *Clostridium argentinense*. The toxins are potentially lethal in very small doses. They act by binding at the neuromuscular junction, blocking nerve transmission and causing flaccid paralysis. Proteolytic strains of *C. botulinum* producing toxin types A, B and F are mesophilic, growing over the range 10–50 °C. Non-proteolytic strains producing toxin types B, E and F are psychrotrophic and can grow at temperatures as low as 3.3 °C. Minimum water activity for growth is 0.93–0.94 and minimum pH for growth is 4.6 (proteolytic strains) or 5.0 (non-proteolytic strains). The toxin is heat-labile and can be destroyed by adequate heat treatment (boiling for 15 minutes). Spores are resistant to normal cooking temperatures, and survive drying and freezing.
Incubation period	Generally 12–36 hours, but may range from a few hours to 8 days.
Symptoms	Vomiting, abdominal pain, fatigue, muscle weakness, headache, dizziness, ocular disturbance (blurred or double vision, dilated pupils, unreactive to light), constipation, dry mouth and difficulty in swallowing and speaking leading ultimately to paralysis and respiratory or heart failure.
Duration	From days up to 8 months; treatment is normally the rapid administration of antitoxin, alkaline stomach washing and mechanical respiratory support.
Reservoir/source	Soil, marine and freshwater sediments and the intestinal tracts of fish, animals, birds and insects.
Mode of transmission and example of foods involved in outbreaks	Ingestion of toxin pre-formed in the food. This may occur when raw or under-processed foods are stored in conditions (temperature, a_w, pH and atmosphere) allowing for growth of the organism. Most outbreaks are due to faulty preservation of food (particularly in homes or cottage industries), e.g. canning, fermentation, curing, smoking, acid or oil preservation. Examples of foods involved include vegetables, condiments (e.g. pepper), fish and fish products (type E), meat and meat products. Several outbreaks have occurred as a result of consumption of uneviscerated fish, garlic in oil

and baked potatoes. Honey is suspected as a mode of transmission of infant botulism.

Specific control measures	The toxin is destroyed by boiling; however, spores require a much higher temperature. *Industrial:* heat sterilization; use of nitrites in pasteurized meat. *Food service establishment/household:* acid-preservation of food at a low pH (<4.6); thorough cooking of home-canned food (boil and stir for 15 minutes); refrigerated storage of food, particularly vacuum-packed, fresh or lightly cured/smoked food. *Consumers* should avoid giving honey or foods containing honey to infants, and discard swollen cans.
Occurrence	Worldwide; particularly frequent among Alaskan populations due to faulty fermentation. Estimated rate of occurrence: +.
Other comments	Case–fatality rate in industrialized countries is in the range 5–10%. In infants, toxicoinfection, infant botulism, may occur and honey is a suspected source.

Type of illness	Brucellosis (undulant fever)
ICD code	ICD-9: 023 ICD-10: A23
Etiological agent	Bacteria: a) *Brucella abortus* b) *Brucella melitensis* c) *Brucella suis*.
Characteristics of the agent	Gram-negative, aerobic, non-spore-forming, short, oval, non-motile rods which grow optimally at 37 °C; heat-labile. Optimum pH for growth: 6.6–7.4.
Incubation period	Variable, from a few days to several weeks or months.
Symptoms	Continuous, intermittent or irregular fever, lassitude, sweat, headache, chills, constipation, body pain, weight loss and anorexia.
Sequelae	Bouts of fever, osteoarticular complications in 20–60% of cases, sacroiliitis, genitourinary complications (including orchitis, epididymitis, sexual impotence), cardiovascular and neurological conditions, insomnia, depression.
Duration	Weeks.
Reservoir/source	Cows, goats, pigs, sheep. a) *Brucella abortus*: cows. b) *Brucella melitensis*: sheep and goats. c) *Brucella suis*: pigs.
Mode of transmission and example of foods involved in outbreaks	Contracted principally from close association with infected animals and therefore an occupational disease of farmers, herdsmen, veterinarians and slaughterhouse workers. It can also be contracted by consumption of milk (usually goat's or sheep's milk), and products made from unpasteurized milk, e.g. fresh goat cheese.
Specific control measures	*Industrial:* heat treatment of milk (pasteurization or sterilization), use of pasteurized milk for cheese production, ageing cheese for at least 90 days. *Food service establishment/household:* heat treatment of milk (boiling). *Other:* vaccination of animals; eradication of diseased animals (testing and slaughtering). *Consumers* should avoid drinking raw milk and eating cheese made with raw milk.

Occurrence	Worldwide, with the exception of parts of northern Europe where it occurs rarely. Incidence in North America is decreasing. Currently reported incidence in the USA is below 120 cases per year. Prevalent in eastern Mediterranean areas, southern Europe, North and East Africa, Central and Southern Asia (India), Central and South America (e.g. Mexico). Estimated rate of occurrence depending on the region: + or ++.
Other comments	The disease is often unrecognized and unreported. Susceptible to antibiotic treatment. Case–fatality rate may be up to 2% if the disease is untreated.

Type of illness	Campylobacteriosis
ICD code	ICD-9: 008.4 ICD-0: A04.5
Etiological agent	Bacteria: *Campylobacter jejuni* and *Campylobacter coli.*
Characteristics of the agent	Gram-negative, non-spore-forming, curved or spiral, motile rods which are sensitive to oxygen and grow best at low oxygen levels in the presence of carbon dioxide. Optimum pH 6.5–7.5. They will not grow below 28–30 °C, grow optimally at 42–45 °C and are very sensitive to heat, salting, reduced pH levels (<6.5) and dry conditions. The organism survives better in chilled conditions than at ambient temperature.
Incubation period	1–11 days, most commonly 2–5 days.
Symptoms	Fever, severe abdominal pain, nausea, and diarrhoea which can vary from slight to profuse watery diarrhoea sometimes containing blood or mucus.
Sequelae	Sequelae may occur in 2–10% of cases. These include reactive arthritis, Guillain–Barré syndrome, haemolytic uraemic syndrome, meningitis, pancreatitis, cholecystitis, colitis, endocarditis, erythema nodosum.
Duration	Up to 10 days; excretion of the organism can continue for 2–3 weeks.
Reservoir/source	Domestic animals (cats, dogs), livestock (pigs, cattle, sheep), birds (poultry), polluted water.
Mode of transmission and example of foods involved in outbreaks	Principally through ingestion of contaminated food. Main food sources are raw milk and raw or undercooked poultry. The bacteria can be spread to other foods by cross-contamination, or contamination with untreated water, contact with animals and birds. Other sources of transmission are contact with live animals (pets and farm animals, e.g. chickens). Person-to-person transmission can also occur during the infectious period which ranges from several days to several weeks. Examples of foods involved include raw milk, poultry, beef, pork and drinking-water.
Specific control measures	*Industrial:* heat treatment (pasteurization/sterilization of milk); hygienic slaughter and processing procedures, irradiation of meat and poultry; treatment of water. *Food service establishment/household:* heat treatment of milk (boiling); thorough cooking of all meat; washing of salads; prevention of cross-contamination of contact surfaces; personal hygiene in food preparation (hand-washing after contact with animals); keeping pets away from food-handling areas.

	Consumers should avoid eating raw or partially cooked poultry and drinking raw milk.
Occurrence	Worldwide. This is one of the most frequently reported foodborne diseases in industrialized countries. In developing countries it is a major cause of infant and traveller's diarrhoea. Some 10–15% of cases of diarrhoeal disease in children, seen at treatment centres, are caused by *Campylobacter* spp. Estimated rate of occurrence: $++/+++$ in industrialized and developing countries respectively.
Other comments	Many infections are asymptomatic. Infected individuals not treated with antibiotics may excrete the organisms for as long as 2–7 weeks. Infection is sometimes misdiagnosed as appendicitis. More sporadic cases occur in the warmer months. The case-fatality rate in industrialized countries is about 0.05%. Infants and young children are the most susceptible.

Type of illness	Cholera
ICD code	ICD-9: 001 ICD-10: A00
Etiological agent	Bacteria: *Vibrio cholerae* 01 (enterotoxin in the gut). Two biotypes are distinguished: classical and eltor. These are further divided into Ogawa and Inaba serotypes. Also, *Vibrio cholerae* 0139.
Characteristics of the agent	Gram-negative, facultatively anaerobic, motile, non-spore-forming rods which grow at 18–42 °C and optimally at 37 °C. Will grow down to a_w 0.97 and over a pH range of 6–11; optimum pH is 7.6. Growth is stimulated by salinity levels of around 3% but is prevented at 6%. The organisms are resistant to freezing but sensitive to heat and acid and may survive for some days on fruit and vegetables. *V. cholerae* is non-invasive and diarrhoea is mediated by cholera toxin formed in the gut.
Incubation period	1–3 days.
Symptoms	Profuse watery diarrhoea, which can lead to severe dehydration, collapse and death within a few hours unless lost fluid and salt are replaced; abdominal pain and vomiting.
Duration	Up to 7 days.
Reservoir/source	Humans. *V. cholerae* is often found in aquatic environments and is part of the normal flora in brackish water and estuaries.
Mode of transmission and example of foods involved in outbreaks	Food and water contaminated through contact with faecal matter of infected food handlers. Contamination of vegetables may occur through sewage or wastewater used for irrigation. Person-to-person transmission through the faecal–oral route is also important. Examples of foods involved include seafood, vegetables, cooked rice, and ice.
Specific control measures	*Industrial*: control measures include safe disposal of excreta and sewage/wastewater; treatment of drinking-water, e.g. chlorination; irradiation, heat treatment of foods, e.g. canning. *Food service establishment/household:* personal hygiene (washing hands with soap and water); thorough cooking of food and careful washing of fruit and vegetables; boiling drinking-water when safe water is not available.

	Consumers should avoid eating raw seafood. In some countries, travellers may need to be vaccinated.
Occurrence	Africa, Asia, parts of Europe and Latin America. In most industrialized countries, reported cholera cases are imported by travellers, or occur as a result of import of food by travellers.
Other comments	In endemic areas, cholera occurs mainly in children because of lack of prior immunity; in epidemics children and adults are equally susceptible. Case–fatality rate can be less than 1% with adequate treatment; in untreated cases, the case–fatality rate may exceed 50%. Estimated rate of occurrence: in industrialized countries cholera occurs rarely and is mainly imported. In Africa and Central and South Africa +/++, and in other parts of the world +.

Type of illness	*Clostridium perfringens* enteritis
ICD code	ICD-9: 005.2 ICD-10: A05.2
Etiological agent	Bacterium: *Clostridium perfringens* (produces enterotoxin in the gut), also known as *Clostridium welchii*.
Characteristics of the agent	Gram-positive, non-motile, anaerobic, spore-forming rods that will grow in the temperature range 12–50 °C, although very slowly below 20 °C. They grow extremely quickly at optimum temperature 43–47 °C. Optimum pH is between 6 and 7, but growth will occur as low as pH 5. Lowest a_w supporting growth is 0.95.
Incubation period	8–24 hours.
Symptoms	Abdominal pain and diarrhoea. Vomiting and fever are rare.
Duration	1–2 days.
Reservoir/source	Soil, sewage, dust, faeces of animals and humans, animal-origin feedstuffs.
Mode of transmission and example of foods involved in outbreaks	Illness is usually caused by cooked meat and poultry dishes subject to time–temperature abuse (i.e. exposure of food to time/temperature conditions permitting bacterial proliferation or not sufficient for reduction of the contaminant(s) to safe levels). The dish has usually been left too long at ambient temperature for cooling before storage, or cooled inadequately. This allows spores surviving the cooking process to germinate and grow, producing large numbers of vegetative cells. If the dish is not reheated sufficiently before consumption to kill the vegetative cells then illness can result. Examples of foods involved include meat and poultry (boiled, stewed).
Specific control measures	*Food service establishment/household:* adequate cooling and cool storage of cooked products: meat-based sauces and large pieces of meat should be cooled to <10 °C within 2–3 hours; thorough reheating of stored food before consumption; preparation of quantities as required when there is no available refrigeration.
Occurrence	Worldwide. Estimated rate of occurrence: ++/+++.
Other comments	Case-fatality rate in industrialized countries is very low at <0.1%.

Type of illness	*Escherichia coli* infections
ICD code	ICD-9: 008.0 ICD-10: A04.0–A04.3 (EPEC: A04.0; ETEC: A04.1, EIEC: A04.2; EHEC: A04.3)
Etiological agent	Bacteria: a) *E. coli* enteropathogenic (EPEC). b) *E. coli* enterotoxigenic (ETEC) produces two types of enterotoxins: a heat-labile toxin (LT) and a heat-stable toxin (ST). c) *E. coli* enteroinvasive (EIEC). d) *E. coli* enterohaemorrhagic (EHEC) or verocytotoxin-producing *E. coli* (VTEC).
Characteristics of the agent	Gram-negative, non-spore-forming, facultatively anaerobic rods, which belong to the family Enterobacteriaceae. Typically mesophile, the bacteria will grow from about 7–10 °C up to 50 °C, with the optimum at 37 °C; in a pH range of 4.4–8.5. Minimum a_w for growth is 0.95. Most *E. coli* spp. are harmless inhabitants of the gut of humans and other warm-blooded animals; however, the strains mentioned above may cause diseases. EHEC is more acid-resistant than other *E. coli*.
Incubation period	a) EPEC: 1–6 days; as short as 12–36 hours. b) ETEC: 1–3 days; as short as 10–12 hours. c) EIEC: 1–3 days; as short as 10–18 hours. d) EHEC: 3–8 days, with a median of 4 days.
Symptoms	a) EPEC infection: enteropathogenic *E. coli* adhere to the gut mucosa and change its absorption capacity causing vomiting, diarrhoea, abdominal pain, and fever. b) ETEC infection: health effects are mediated by enterotoxins. Symptoms include diarrhoea (ranging from mild afebrile diarrhoea to a severe, cholera-like syndrome of profuse diarrhoea without blood or mucus), abdominal cramps and vomiting, sometimes leading to dehydration and shock. c) EIEC infection: inflammatory disease of the gut mucosa and submucosa caused by the invasion and multiplication of EIEC in the epithelial cells of the colon. Symptoms include fever, severe abdominal pain, vomiting and watery diarrhoea (in <10% of cases stools may become bloody and may contain mucus). d) EHEC infection: abdominal cramps, watery diarrhoea that may develop into bloody diarrhoea (haemorrhagic colitis). Fever and vomiting may also occur.
Sequelae	EPEC, ETEC, EIEC infections are an underlying factor of malnutrition in infants and children in developing countries.

EHEC infections may result in life-threatening complications, such as haemolytic uraemic syndrome (HUS), in up to 10% of patients, particularly young children and the elderly. HUS is characterized by acute renal failure, haemolytic anaemia and thrombocytopenia. Other sequelae include erythema nodosum and thrombotic thrombocytopenic purpura.

Duration	a) EPEC: days–weeks. b) ETEC: up to 5 days. c) EIEC: days–weeks. d) EHEC: days–weeks.
Reservoir/source	Humans are the main reservoir for EPEC, ETEC, EIEC. The reservoir for EHEC is mainly cattle.
Mode of transmission and example of foods involved in outbreaks	a–c) EPEC, ETEC, EIEC infections: consumption of food and water contaminated with faecal matter. Time–temperature abuse of such food increases the risk of illness. Up to 25% of infections in infants and young children in developing countries are due to *E. coli*, in particular ETEC and EPEC, which are observed in 10–20% and 1–5% of cases at treatment centres respectively. ETEC is also a major cause of traveller's diarrhoea in developing countries. d) EHEC infection is transmitted mainly through consumption of foods such as raw or undercooked ground-meat products, and raw milk, from infected animals. Faecal contamination of water and other foods, as well as cross-contamination during food preparation, will also lead to infection. Examples of foods involved include ground (minced) meat, raw milk, and vegetables. Secondary transmission (person-to-person) may also occur during the period of excretion which is less than a week for adults but up to 3 weeks in one-third of children affected.
Specific control measures	*Industrial:* treatment of drinking-water, and an effective sewage disposal system. *Food service establishment/household:* specific control measures based on prevention of direct and indirect contamination of food and water with faecal matter; thorough cooking and reheating of food; and good personal hygiene. For EHEC infection, control measures include: *Industrial:* irradiation of meat, or thorough heat processing of meat; pasteurization/sterilization of milk; treatment of wastewater used for irrigation. *Food service establishment/household:* thorough cooking of meat, boiling of milk or use of pasteurized milk; hand-washing before preparation of food.

	Consumers should avoid eating raw or partially cooked meat and poultry and drinking raw milk.
Occurrence	Worldwide. *E. coli* infections are highly prevalent in developing countries where the estimated rate of occurrence is +++. EHEC infections are mainly reported in Argentina, Chile, Europe (France, Germany, Italy, Sweden, UK), Japan and North America.
Other comments	The case–fatality rate of EPEC, ETEC, EIEC infections in industrialized countries is estimated to be less than 0.1%. The case–fatality rate of EHEC infection is about 2%. The fatality rate of *E. coli* infections in infants and children is much higher in developing countries. Children and the elderly are particularly vulnerable to this infection and may suffer more severely. The majority of cases of EHEC infections are reported in summer.

Type of illness	Listeriosis
ICD code	ICD-9: 027 ICD-10: A32
Etiological agent	Bacterium: *Listeria monocytogenes.*
Characteristics of the agent	Gram-positive, non-spore-forming, facultatively anaerobic rods. Psychrotrophic, capable of growing in a temperature range of 3–42 °C, but optimally at about 30–35 °C. The pH range for growth is 5.0–9.0. Minimum pH and a_w for growth are 4.4 and 0.92 respectively. The bacteria are able to grow in the presence of 10% salt.
Incubation period	A few days to several weeks.
Symptoms	Influenza-like symptoms such as fever, headache and occasionally gastrointestinal symptoms.
Sequelae	Meningoencephalitis and/or septicaemia in newborns and adults and abortion in pregnant women. The onset of meningoencephalitis (rare in pregnant women) may be sudden with fever, intense headaches, nausea, vomiting and signs of meningeal irritation. Delirium and coma may appear early; occasionally there is collapse and shock.
Duration	Days–weeks.
Reservoir/source	Water, soil, sewage, sludge, decaying vegetables, silage and faeces of numerous wild and domestic animals. Other sources may be infected animals and people.
Mode of transmission and example of foods involved in outbreaks	A substantial proportion of cases of listeriosis are foodborne. Examples of foods involved include raw milk, soft cheese, meat-based paste, jellied pork tongue, raw vegetables and coleslaw.
Specific control measures	*Industrial:* heat treatment of milk (pasteurization, sterilization) with measures to ensure reduction of processing contamination risks. For ready-to-eat high-risk processed foods, reduction of all cross-contamination risks after processing. *Food service establishment/household:* use of pasteurized or heat-treated (boiled) milk and products made from pasteurized or heat-treated milk; refrigeration of perishable foods and consumption within a short space of time. Pre-cooked refrigerated foods should be thoroughly reheated before consumption. Avoidance of certain high-risk foods, e.g. soft cheese, ready-to-eat meat such as meat paste, and raw milk and raw milk products during pregnancy.

	Consumers, particularly pregnant women and other vulnerable individuals, should avoid eating raw foods of animal origin, e.g. raw meat, raw milk. Pregnant women should also avoid foods which support growth of *Listeria*, e.g. soft cheese, pre-prepared salad, cold, smoked or raw seafood, paté.
Occurrence	Estimated rate of occurrence: +. The majority of cases reported have been from Europe, North America and the islands of the Pacific.
Other comments	The most severe form of illness occurs in fetuses and neonates, the elderly and those who are immunocompromised. About one-third of clinical cases occur in the newborn. In adults infection occurs mainly in those aged 40 or over. Transplacental fetal infection may lead to abortion or stillbirth. Asymptomatic infection may occur at all ages. Infected individuals may shed the organisms in their stools for several months. Case-fatality rate is up to 30%; in patients who have not received adequate treatment the case-fatality rate may be as high as 70%. Pregnant women and fetuses, the elderly, and immunocompromised individuals, including those receiving treatments for cancer, are the most susceptible.

Type of illness	Salmonellosis
ICD code	ICD-9: 003 ICD-10: A02.0
Etiological agent	Bacteria: non-typhoid *Salmonella* serotypes.
Characteristics of the agent	Gram-negative, mesophilic, facultatively anaerobic, motile, non-spore-forming rods. Growth can occur between 5 °C and 47 °C. Optimum growth occurs at 37 °C. Minimum pH and a_w for growth are 4 and 0.95 respectively.
Incubation period	6–48 hours, occasionally up to 4 days.
Symptoms	The principal symptoms are fever, headache, nausea, vomiting, abdominal pain and diarrhoea.
Sequelae	Reactive arthritis, septicaemia, aortitis, cholecystitis, colitis, meningitis, myocarditis, osteomyelitis, pancreatitis, Reiter disease, rheumatoid syndromes.
Duration	Usually a few days to 1 week, but sometimes infection may last up to 3 weeks.
Reservoir/source	A wide range of domestic and wild animals, including poultry, pigs, cattle, rodents, iguanas, tortoises, turtles, and pets such as dogs and cats. Also humans, i.e. patients and convalescent carriers.
Mode of transmission and example of foods involved in outbreaks	The main route of transmission is by ingestion of the organisms in food (milk, meat, poultry, eggs) derived from infected food animals. Food can also be contaminated by infected food handlers, pets and pests, or by cross-contamination owing to poor hygiene. Contamination of food and water may also occur from the faeces of an infected animal or person. Problems caused by initial contamination may be exacerbated by prolonged storage at temperatures at which the organism may grow. Direct person-to-person transmission may also occur during the course of the infection. Examples of foods involved include unpasteurized milk, raw eggs, poultry, meat, spices, salads, chocolate.
Specific control measures	*Industrial:* effective heat-processing of foods of animal origin including pasteurization of milk and eggs; irradiation of meat and poultry. *Food service establishment/household:* safe food preparation practices, including thorough cooking and reheating of food and boiling of milk; adequate refrigeration; prevention of cross-contamination, cleaning and disinfection of food preparation surfaces; exclusion of pets and other animals from food-handling areas.

	Consumers, particularly vulnerable groups, should avoid raw and undercooked meat and poultry, as well as raw milk and raw eggs and foods containing raw eggs.
Occurrence	Worldwide. Estimated rate of occurrence: $++/+++$. A drastic increase in incidence of salmonellosis, due particularly to *S. enteritidis*, has occurred during the past two decades in Europe, North America and some other countries. In Europe and North America, contaminated eggs and poultry have been the major source of infection.
Other comments	General susceptibility is increased by achlorhydria, antacid therapy, immunosuppressive therapy and debilitating conditions, including malnutrition. The severity of the illness is related to serotype, the number of organisms ingested and host factors. Case–fatality rate is less than 1% in industrialized countries. Symptomless excretion of the organism can continue for several weeks or, in some cases, months.

Type of illness	Shigellosis (or bacillary dysentery)
ICD code	ICD-9: 004 ICD-10: A03
Etiological agent	Bacteria: *Shigella dysenteriae, S. flexneri, S. boydii, S. sonnei.*
Characteristics of the agent	Gram-negative, non-motile, non-spore-forming, facultatively anaerobic rods. Typically mesophilic: growing between 10 °C and 45 °C and optimally at 37 °C. The bacteria grow best in the pH range 6–8 and do not survive below pH 4.5. The minimum a_w for growth is 0.97.
Incubation period	1–3 days, up to 1 week for *S. dysenteriae.*
Symptoms	Abdominal pain, vomiting, fever accompanied by diarrhoea that can range from watery (*S. sonnei*) to a dysenteric syndrome of bloody stools containing mucus and pus (*S. dysenteriae* and, to a lesser extent, *S. flexneri* and *S. boydii*).
Sequelae	In 2–3% of cases these may be: haemolytic uraemic syndrome, erythema nodosum, Reiter disease, splenic abscesses, synovitis.
Duration	A few days to a few weeks.
Reservoir/source	Humans.
Mode of transmission and example of foods involved in outbreaks	Food and water contaminated with faecal matter. Person-to-person transmission through the faecal–oral route is an important mode of transmission. Food can be contaminated by food handlers with poor personal hygiene or by use of sewage/wastewater for fertilization. Examples of foods involved include uncooked foods that have received extensive handling such as mixed salads and vegetables; water and raw milk.
Specific control measures	*Industrial:* treatment of drinking-water and an effective sewage disposal system. *Food service establishment/household:* safe food preparation practices including careful hand-washing with soap and water, thorough cooking and reheating of food prior to consumption, disinfection of food preparation surfaces and thorough washing of all fruit and vegetables.
Occurrence	Worldwide, with a higher prevalence in developing countries. Shigellosis is a major cause of diarrhoea in infants and children under the age of 5 years, and constitutes 5–15% of diarrhoeal disease cases seen at treatment centres. *S. dysenteriae* type 1 has been responsible for large epidemics of severe dysentery in Central America and recently Central Africa and southern Asia.

	Depending on the degree of development the estimated rate of occurrence may vary between + and +++.
Other comments	In developing countries, *S. flexneri* is the most common cause of infection. However, *S. dysenteriae* type 1, occurring in epidemic regions, causes the most severe disease. In industrialized countries, *S. sonnei* is the most common species isolated, and milder illness is the norm.
	The disease is more severe in young children than in adults among whom many infections may be asymptomatic. The elderly and those suffering from malnutrition are particularly susceptible and may develop severe symptoms or even die. Travellers are particularly at risk.
	Case-fatality rate in industrialized countries is low and estimated at 0.1%.

Type of illness	*Staphylococcus aureus* intoxication
ICD code	ICD-9: 005.0 ICD-10: A05.0
Etiological agent	Bacterial toxin: *Staphylococcus aureus* enterotoxin.
Characteristics of the agent	Gram-positive, non-motile, non-spore-forming, facultatively anaerobic cocci. Growth temperature is between 7 °C and 48 °C, with an optimum of about 37 °C. The bacteria grow in a pH range of 4.0–9.3. Optimum pH is 7.0–7.5. The range over which enterotoxin is produced is narrower, with little toxin production below pH 6.0. Growth will occur down to an a_w of 0.83, but toxin production does not occur below 0.86. This is the most resistant bacterial pathogen with regard to decreased water activity. Intoxication is caused by a toxin which is formed in the food. The toxin is relatively heat-stable and can survive boiling for more than an hour. It is therefore possible for well-cooked food to cause illness but not contain any viable *S. aureus* cells.
Incubation period	2–6 hours
Symptoms	An intoxication, sometimes of abrupt and violent onset. Severe nausea, cramps, vomiting and prostration, sometimes accompanied by diarrhoea.
Duration	About 2 days.
Reservoir/source	Humans (skin, nose, throat). *S. aureus* is carried by about 25–40% of the healthy population.
Mode of transmission and example of foods involved in outbreaks	Consumption of foods containing the toxin. Foods are contaminated by food handlers. If storage conditions are inadequate, the bacteria may multiply to produce toxin. Intoxication is often associated with cooked food, e.g. meat, where competitive bacteria have been destroyed. Examples of foods involved include prepared foods subject to handling in their preparation (ham, chicken and egg salads, cream-filled products, ice-cream, cheese).
Specific control measures	*Food service establishment/household*: Exclusion of food handlers with visibly infected skin lesions (boils, cuts etc.) from work; thorough personal hygiene of workers; prevention of time–temperature abuse in handling cooked/ready-to-eat foods.
Occurrence	Worldwide. The estimated rate of occurrence varies between ++ and +++ depending on conditions of food hygiene.
Other comments	Case–fatality rate is estimated at less than 0.02%.

Type of illness	Typhoid and paratyphoid fevers
ICD code	ICD-9: 002.0 and 002.1–002.9 ICD-10: A01.0 and A01.1–A01.4
Etiological agent	Bacteria: *Salmonella typhi* and *Salmonella paratyphi* types A–C.
Characteristics of the agent	As for non-typhoid salmonellae, except minimum growth pH is higher (4.9).
Incubation period	10–20 days with a range of 3 days to 8 weeks.
Symptoms	Systemic infections characterized by high fever, abdominal pains, headache, vomiting, diarrhoea followed by constipation, rashes and other symptoms of generalized infection.
Sequelae	Haemolytic anaemia.
Duration	Several weeks to months.
Reservoir/source	Humans.
Mode of transmission and example of foods involved in outbreaks	Ingestion of food and water contaminated with faecal matter. Food handlers carrying the pathogen may be an important source of food contamination. Secondary transmission may also occur. Examples of foods involved include prepared foods, dairy products (e.g. raw milk), meat products, shellfish, vegetables, salads.
Specific control measures	*Industrial:* treatment of drinking-water, and an effective sewage disposal system. *Food service establishment/household:* safe food preparation practices including careful hand-washing with soap and water, thorough cooking and reheating of food prior to consumption, disinfection of food preparation surfaces and thorough washing of all fruit and vegetables.
Occurrence	Predominantly in developing countries where the estimated rate of occurrence is ++. In industrialized countries the estimated rate of occurrence is +.
Other comments	Excretion of the organism may occur after recovery or by asymptomatic carriers, and this may be lifelong unless treated. Case–fatality rate is estimated at about 6% in industrialized countries.

Type of illness	*Vibrio parahaemolyticus* gastroenteritis
ICD code	ICD-9: 005.4 ICD-10: A.05.3
Etiological agent	Bacterium: *Vibrio parahaemolyticus.*
Characteristics of the agent	Basic characteristics are the same as for *V. cholerae. V. parahaemolyticus* differs in that it is more halophilic and will grow at salt levels up to 8% and with a minimum a_w of 0.94. Growth is optimal and very fast at 37 °C (doubling time about 10 minutes) and will occur down to around 10 °C. *V. parahaemolyticus* is more sensitive to extremes of temperature than *V. cholerae* and will die at chill temperatures.
Incubation period	Often 9–25 hours, up to 3 days.
Symptoms	Profuse watery diarrhoea free from blood or mucus, abdominal pain, vomiting, and fever. A dysenteric syndrome has been reported from some countries, particularly Japan.
Sequelae	Septicaemia.
Duration	Up to 8 days.
Reservoir/source	Natural habitat is coastal seawater and estuarine brackish waters above 15 °C, and marine fish and shellfish.
Mode of transmission and example of foods involved in outbreaks	Mainly consumption of raw or undercooked fish and fishery products, or cooked foods subject to cross-contamination from raw fish.
Specific control measures	*Food service establishment/household:* thorough heat treatment of seafood; rapid chilling; prevention of cross-contamination from raw seafood products to other foods or preparation surfaces.
Occurrence	The illness has been reported primarily in countries in the WHO Western Pacific Region and in particular Japan as well as the WHO South-East Asia Region and the USA. Estimated rate of occurrence: +/++.
Other comments	Case–fatality rate in industrialized countries is less than 1%.

Type of illness	*Vibrio vulnificus* infection
ICD code	ICD-9: 005.8 ICD-10: A05.8
Etiological agent	Bacterium: *Vibrio vulnificus*.
Characteristics of the agent	Gram-negative, non-spore-forming rods. Optimal temperature for growth is 37 °C.
Incubation period	12 hours–3 days.
Symptoms	Profuse diarrhoea with blood in stools; the organism is associated with wound infections and septicaemia which may originate from the gastrointestinal tract, or traumatized epithelial surfaces.
Sequelae	Produces septicaemia in persons with chronic liver diseases, chronic alcohol dependence, haemochromatosis, or those who are immunodepressed. Over 50% of patients with primary septicaemia may die; the fatality rate increases to 90% in hypotensive individuals.
Duration	Days–weeks.
Reservoir/source	Natural habitat is coastal or estuarine waters.
Mode of transmission and example of foods involved in outbreaks	All known cases are associated with seafood, particularly raw oysters.
Specific control measures	*Consumers*, particularly vulnerable groups including the elderly, those with underlying liver disease or immunodepressed through treatment or disease, and alcohol-dependent persons, should not eat raw seafood.
Occurrence	Frequently in Europe, USA and the WHO Western Pacific Region. Estimated rate of occurrence: +/++.
Other comments	Case–fatality rate can be as high as 40–60%.

Type of illness	Yersiniosis
ICD code	ICD-9: 027.8 ICD-10: A04.6
Etiological agent	Bacterium: *Yersinia enterocolitica*.
Characteristics of the agent	Gram-negative, facultatively anaerobic, motile, non-spore-forming rods of the family Enterobacteriaceae. *Y. enterocolitica* is a psychrotroph capable of growing at temperatures between 0 °C and 44 °C, but optimally at 29 °C. Growth will occur in a pH range of 4.6–9.0, but optimally at pH 7–8. It will grow in media containing 5% salt but not 7% salt.
Incubation period	1–11 days (but usually 24–36 hours).
Symptoms	Abdominal pain, diarrhoea accompanied by a mild fever, and sometimes vomiting.
Sequelae	Sequelae are observed in 2–3% of cases: reactive arthritis, Reiter disease, eye complaints and rash, cholangitis, erythema nodosum, septicaemia, hepatic and splenic abscesses, lymphadenitis, pneumonia, spondylitis.
Duration	Symptoms usually abate after 2–3 days; although they may continue in a milder form for 1–3 weeks.
Reservoir/source	A variety of animals, but pathogenic strains are most frequently isolated from pigs.
Mode of transmission and example of foods involved in outbreaks	Illness is transmitted through consumption of pork products (tongue, tonsils, gut), cured or uncured, as well as milk and milk products.
Specific control measures	*Food service establishment/household:* thorough cooking of pork products, and prevention of cross-contamination.
Occurrence	Northern Europe and Australia: estimated rate of occurrence: +/++; USA: estimated rate of occurrence: +.
Other comments	Untreated cases continue to excrete the organism for 2–3 months. The disease is often misdiagnosed as appendicitis. Case–fatality rate is 0.03%.

Type of illness	Viral gastroenteriti
ICD code	ICD-9: 008.8 ICD-10: A08
Etiological agent	Viruses: a number of different viruses have been established as causes of gastroenteritis. These include adenoviruses, coronaviruses, rotaviruses, parvoviruses, caliciviruses and astroviruses. Those most commonly associated with foodborne outbreaks are described as small, round, structured viruses (SRSV), which include Norwalk agent.
Characteristics of the agent	These viruses exhibit a range of biochemical and physical characteristics.
Incubation period	15–50 hours.
Symptoms	Diarrhoea, and vomiting which is often severe and projectile with sudden onset.
Duration	2 days.
Reservoir/source	Humans.
Mode of transmission and example of foods involved in outbreaks	Gastroenteritis viruses are usually spread by the faecal–oral route. Food and drinking-water may be contaminated either at source when exposed to sewage/wastewater in the environment or used for irrigation, or by an infected food handler. Filter-feeding shellfish are the most common food contaminated at source, but a far wider range of different cooked and uncooked foods have been implicated in secondary contamination by food handlers.
Specific control measures	Hygienic sewage disposal, treatment of drinking-water, treatment of wastewater used for irrigation. Good personal hygiene (i.e. hand hygiene); abstinence from handling food when ill, especially when diarrhoea is present.
Occurrence	Worldwide. Estimated rate of occurrence for rotavirus: $++/+++$; and for other viral infections: $+$. Rotavirus infections constitute 15–25% of diarrhoeal disease cases identified in children and seen at treatment centres in the developing countries.

Type of illness	Viral hepatitis A
ICD code	ICD-9: 070.1 ICD-10: B15
Etiological agent	Virus: hepatitis A virus (member of Picornaviridae).
Characteristics of the agent	Small round virus, about 28 nm in diameter, containing single-stranded RNA. The virus multiplies in the gut epithelium before being carried by the blood to the liver. In the later part of incubation, the virus is shed in the faeces. Relatively acid-resistant.
Incubation period	2–6 weeks; usually about 25 days.
Symptoms	Early symptoms are loss of appetite, fever, malaise, abdominal discomfort, nausea and vomiting. These are followed by signs of liver damage such as passage of dark urine, pale stools and jaundice.
Sequelae	Liver disorders, particularly in older persons.
Duration	Varies in clinical severity: mild, with recovery within few weeks, to severe, lasting several months.
Reservoir/source	Humans: sewage and contaminated water.
Mode of transmission and example of foods involved in outbreaks	Spread through the faecal–oral route, primarily person-to-person. It can also be transmitted through food and water as a result of sewage contamination or infected food handlers. Risk of transmission is greatest during the second half of the incubation period until a few days after the appearance of jaundice. Examples of foods involved include: shellfish, raw fruit and vegetables, bakery products.
Specific control measures	*Industrial:* treatment of water supply, safe sewage disposal. *Food service establishment/household:* good personal hygiene, in particular, thorough hand-washing with soap and water before handling foods and abstinence from handling food when infected; thorough cooking of shellfish. An effective vaccine is available, and vaccination of professional food handlers and travellers should be considered.
Occurrence	Worldwide. Estimated rate of occurrence: ++.
Other comments	There may be asymptomatic carriers. Infection in adults is most severe. In children it is often asymptomatic and confers immunity. Case-fatality rate is low, about 0.3%. A higher case-fatality rate may occur in adults over 50 years of age.

Type of illness	Poliomyelitis
ICD code	ICD-9: 045 ICD-10: A80
Etiological agent	Virus: poliovirus; member of Picornaviridae.
Characteristics of the agent	Small round virus, which contains single-stranded RNA and can withstand acidity in the range of pH 3–5. The poliovirus infects the gastrointestinal tract and spreads to the regional nodes, and, in a minority of cases, to the nervous system.
Incubation period	3–14 days.
Symptoms	Poliomyelitis may be a transient viraemia characterized by fever and malaise. In a minority of cases, it may progress to a second stage of persistent viraemia where the virus invades the central nervous system causing varying degrees of paralysis and in some cases even death. Severe muscle pain and stiffness of the neck and back with or without flaccid paralysis are symptoms of the more severe illness. Flaccid paralysis occurs in less than 1% of poliovirus infections. Most often paralysis is in the legs, sometimes in the arms. Paralysis of the muscles used in respiration and/or swallowing is life-threatening. The infection in young children is usually asymptomatic and confers immunity, but is more severe in older children and young adults.
Sequelae	Permanent paralysis.
Reservoir/source	Humans; most frequently people with no apparent symptoms of infection.
Mode of transmission and example of foods involved in outbreaks	Principally person-to-person, through the faecal–oral route. Food and drinking-water are potential modes of transmission where hygiene standards are low. In some instances, milk and other foodstuffs contaminated with faeces have been a vehicle for transmission.
Specific control measures	Vaccination. Specific control measures with regard to food include: *Industrial:* treatment of drinking-water, and an effective sewage disposal system. *Food service establishment/household:* safe food preparation practices including careful hand-washing with soap and water, thorough cooking and reheating of food prior to consumption and thorough washing of all fruit and vegetables.
Occurrence	Poliomyelitis has been almost entirely eradicated in industrialized countries and the Americas as a result of effective immunization. In

	developing countries the estimated rate of occurrence varies from + to ++, depending on immunization programmes.
Other comments	During the few days prior to, and following the onset of symptoms, the risk of transmission is greatest. Infants and children under 5 years of age are the most frequently affected. Immunization of the elderly is recommended, particularly when travelling abroad.

Type of illness	Amoebiasis (amoebic dysentery)
ICD code	ICD-9: 006 ICD-10: A06
Etiological agent	Protozoa: *Entamoeba histolytica*.
Characteristics of the agent	An amoeboid protozoa that is an aerotolerant anaerobe. It survives in the environment in an encysted form. Cysts remain viable and infective for several days in faeces and may survive in soil for at least 8 days at 28–34 °C, and for more than 1 month at 10 °C. Relatively resistant to chlorine.
Incubation period	2–4 weeks, but may range from a few days to several months.
Symptoms	Severe bloody diarrhoea, stomach pains, fever and vomiting. Most infections remain symptomless.
Sequelae	Liver abscess.
Duration	Weeks–months.
Reservoir/source	Mainly humans, but also dogs and rats. The organism is also found in nightsoil, and sewage irrigation.
Mode of transmission and example of foods involved in outbreaks	Transmission occurs mainly through the ingestion of faecally contaminated food and water containing cysts. Cysts are excreted in large numbers (up to 5×10^7 cysts per day) by an infected individual. Illness is spread by the faecal–oral route, person-to-person contact or faecally contaminated food and water. Examples of foods involved include fruit and vegetables, and drinking-water.
Specific control measures	*Industrial:* filtration and disinfection of water supply; hygienic disposal of sewage water, treatment of irrigation water. *Food service establishment/household:* boiling of water, when safe water is not available; thorough washing of fruit and vegetables; thorough cooking of food; good hand hygiene.
Occurrence	Worldwide, particularly in young adults. Estimated rate of occurrence: very low in industrialized countries: +; very high in developing countries with poor sanitation: ++.

Type of illness	Cryptosporidiosis
ICD code	ICD-9: 136.8 ICD-10: A07.2
Etiological agent	Protozoa: *Cryptosporidium parvum.*
Characteristics of the agent	The organism has a complex life cycle that can take place in a single human or animal host. It produces resistant oocysts, typically 4–6 μm, which are very resistant to the chlorination process, but are killed by conventional cooking procedures.
Incubation period	2–14 days.
Symptoms	Diarrhoea (persistent diarrhoea), nausea, vomiting and abdominal pain sometimes accompanied by an influenza-like illness and fever.
Sequelae	Illness is more serious in the immunocompromised, particularly AIDS patients, and leads to severe nutrient malabsorption and weight loss.
Duration	A few days up to 3 weeks.
Reservoir/source	Humans and wild and domestic animals, e.g. cattle.
Mode of transmission and example of foods involved in outbreaks	Spread through the faecal–oral route, person-to-person contact, or consumption of faecally contaminated food and water. Other routes of transmission include swallowing water in contaminated swimming pools. Examples of foods involved include raw milk, drinking-water and apple cider.
Specific control measures	*Industrial:* pasteurization/sterilization of milk, filtration and disinfection of water, sanitary disposal of excreta, sewage and wastewater. *Food service establishment/household:* boiling of water when safe water is not available; boiling of milk; thorough cooking of food; good hand hygiene.
Occurrence	Worldwide. Cryptosporidiosis is one of the leading causes of diarrhoeal disease in infants and young children. It constitute 5–15% of diarrhoeal disease cases in children seen at treatment centres. The estimated occurrence is +++. In industrialized countries, it occurs often in day-care centres. Estimated occurrence: ++.
Other comments	Children under the age of 5 years are more at risk. Immunocompromised individuals, e.g. AIDS patients, may suffer from longer and more severe infection. In AIDS patients, infection may lead to death.

Type of illness	Giardiasis
ICD code	ICD-9: 007.1 ICD-10: A.07.1
Etiological agent	Protozoan: *Giardia lamblia.*
Characteristics of the agent	This flagellate protozoan has an environmentally resistant cyst stage as well as the vegetative trophozoite stage. Cysts are oval and 7–14 μm long. They are resistant to the chlorination process used in most water-treatment systems but are killed by conventional cooking procedures.
Incubation period	4–25 days, usually 7–10 days.
Symptoms	Once ingested the cysts release the active trophozoite which adheres to the gut wall. Illness is characterized by diarrhoea (which may be chronic and relapsing), abdominal cramps, fatigue, weight loss, anorexia and nausea. It is thought that the symptoms may be caused by a protein toxin.
Sequelae	Cholangitis, dystrophy, lymphoid hyperplasia.
Duration	Weeks–years.
Reservoir/source	Humans and animals.
Mode of transmission and example of foods involved in outbreaks	*Giardia* cysts are excreted in large numbers by an infected individual. Illness is spread through the faecal–oral route, person-to-person contact or faecally contaminated food and water. Cysts have been isolated from lettuces and fruit such as strawberries. The infection is also associated with drinking-water from surface waters and shallow wells. Examples of foods involved include: water, home-canned salmon and noodle salad.
Specific control measures	*Industrial:* filtration and disinfection of water supply; sanitary disposal of excreta and sewage; treatment of irrigation water. *Food service establishment/household:* boiling of water, when safe water is not available; thorough washing of fruit and vegetables; thorough cooking of foods; good hand hygiene. *Consumers,* such as campers, should avoid drinking surface water unless it has been boiled or filtered.
Occurrence	Worldwide. In industrialized countries, the estimated rate of occurrence is ++ and in developing countries with poor sanitation +++.
Other comments	Number of asymptomatic carriers is high. Children are affected more frequently than adults. Illness is prolonged and more serious in the immunocompromised, particularly AIDS patients. Tourists are particularly at risk.

Type of illness	Toxoplasmosis and congenital toxoplasmosis
ICD code	ICD-9: 130 and 771.2 ICD-10: B58 and P 37.1
Etiological agent	Protozoan: *Toxoplasma gondii* (belonging to the family Sarcocystidae).
Characteristics of the agent	A coccidian protozoan.
Incubation period	5–23 days.
Symptoms	Infections are often asymptomatic or present an acute disease with lymphadenopathy and lymphocytosis persisting for days or weeks.
Sequelae	During pregnancy transplacental infection may cause abortion or stillbirth, chorioretinitis, brain damage. In immunocompromised individuals infection may cause cerebritis, chorioretinitis, pneumonia, myocarditis, rash, or/and death. Cerebral toxoplasmosis is a particular threat for AIDS patients.
Reservoir/source	Cats and other felines; intermediate hosts are sheep, goats, rodents, pigs, cattle and birds, all of which may carry an infective stage of *T. gondii* encysted in tissue, e.g. muscle or brain, which remains viable for long periods, perhaps the entire life of the animal.
Mode of transmission and example of foods involved in outbreaks	Infections occur through ingestion of oocysts. Children may acquire the infection by playing in sand polluted with cat excreta. Oocysts shed by cats can sporulate and become infective 1–5 days later and may remain infective in water or soil for a year. Infection may also be acquired by eating raw or undercooked meat containing the cysts or food and water contaminated with feline faeces. Transplacental infection may also occur when the infection is acquired during pregnancy. Examples of foods involved include raw or undercooked meat, vegetables and goat's milk.
Specific control measures	*Industrial:* irradiation of meat. *Food service establishments, household:* thorough cooking of meat; careful washing of fruits and vegetables; good personal hygiene—particularly after contact with cats and before food preparation: safe disposal of cat faeces. *Consumers,* particularly pregnant women if not immune, should be advised to avoid raw or undercooked meat, wash vegetables carefully and wash hands after contact with cats.
Occurrence	Worldwide. Estimated rate of occurrence: + to ++.

Other comments	*T. gondii* cysts remain in the tissue and may reactivate if the immune system becomes compromised, e.g. by cytotoxic or immunosuppressive therapy or in patients with AIDS. In these groups the infection may be fulminant and fatal.

Type of illness	Anisakiasis
ICD code	ICD-9: 127.1 ICD-10: B81.0
Etiological agent	Helminth (nematode/roundworm): *Anisakis* spp. (larval stage).
Characteristics of the agent	Slender, threadlike parasite measuring 15–16 mm in length and 1 mm in diameter.
Incubation period	A few hours; symptoms related to the intestine a few days or weeks.
Symptoms	The motile larvae burrow into the stomach wall producing acute ulceration and nausea, vomiting and epigastric pain, sometimes with haematemesis. They migrate upward and attach themselves to the oropharynx causing coughing. In the small intestine they cause eosinophilic abscesses.
Reservoir/source	Sea mammals (for *Anisakis* spp. that are parasitic to humans).
Mode of transmission and example of foods involved in outbreaks	Consumption of the muscles of certain saltwater fish that have been inadequately processed. Examples of foods involved include sushi, sashimi, herring, cebiche.
Specific control measures	*Industrial:* irradiation; heat treatment, freezing, candling, cleaning (evisceration) of fish as soon as possible after they are caught (will prevent post-mortem migration of infective larvae from the mesenteries of the fish to muscles). *Food service establishment/household:* cleaning of fish; thorough cooking before consumption; freezing (−23 °C for 7 days).
Occurrence	Mainly in countries where consumption of raw or inadequately processed fish is common, e.g. Northern Europe, Japan, Latin America. Over 12 000 cases have been reported in Japan. Cases have also been reported in other parts of the world as eating habits change with migration.
Other comments	Symptoms mimic those of appendicitis.

Type of illness	Ascariasis
ICD code	ICD-9: 127.0 ICD-10: B77
Etiological agent	Helminth (nematode/roundworm): *Ascaris lumbricoides* (egg with infective larva).
Characteristics of the agent	*Ascaris lumbricoides* is a large roundworm infecting the small intestine. Adult males are 15–31 cm × 2–4 mm and females are 20–40 cm × 3–6 mm. Eggs undergo embryonation in the soil; after 2–3 weeks at warm temperature they become infective and may remain viable for several months or even years in favourable soils. The larvae emerge from the egg in the duodenum, penetrate the intestinal wall and reach the heart and the lungs in the blood. Larvae grow and develop in the lungs; 9–10 days after infection they break out of the pulmonary capillaries into the alveoli and migrate through the bronchial tubes and trachea into the pharynx where they are swallowed and reach the intestine 14–20 days after infection. In the intestine they develop into adults and begin laying eggs 40–60 days after ingestion of the embryonated eggs. The life cycle is complete after 8 weeks.
Incubation period	First appearance of eggs in stools is 60–70 days. In larval ascariasis, symptoms occur 4–16 days after infection.
Symptoms	Gastrointestinal discomfort, colic and vomiting, fever; observation of live worms in stools. Some patients may have pulmonary symptoms or neurological disorders during migration of the larvae. However, there are generally few or no symptoms.
Sequelae	A heavy worm infestation may cause nutritional deficiency; other complications, sometimes fatal, include obstruction of the bowel by a bolus of worms (observed particularly in children), obstruction of bile or pancreatic duct.
Reservoir/source	Humans; soil and vegetation on which faecal matter containing eggs has been deposited.
Mode of transmission and example of foods involved in outbreaks	Ingestion of infective eggs from soil contaminated with human faeces or from contaminated vegetables and water.
Specific control measures	Use of toilet facilities; safe excreta disposal; protection of food from dirt and soil; thorough washing of produce. Food dropped on the floor should not be eaten without washing or cooking, particularly in endemic areas.
Occurrence	Worldwide. There is a high prevalence (exceeding 50%) in moist and tropical countries. Estimated rate of occurrence: + to +++ depending on the region.
Other comments	In endemic areas the highest prevalence is among children aged 3–8 years.

Type of illness	Trichinellosis (trichiniasis, trichinosis)
ICD code	ICD-9: 124 ICD-10: B75
Etiological agent	Helminth (nematode/roundworm): *Trichinella spiralis* (larvae in infected muscle).
Characteristics of the agent	White intestinal worm, visible to the naked eye. The transmissible form of this parasite is a larval cyst approximately 0.4 mm × 0.25 mm which occurs in pork muscle. In the initial phase of trichinellosis, the larvae ingested with the meat develop rapidly into adults in the epithelium of the intestine. Female worms produce larvae which penetrate the lymphatics or venules and are disseminated via the blood throughout the body. The larvae become encapsulated in the skeletal muscle.
Incubation period	Initial phase: a few days. Systemic symptoms: 8–21 days.
Symptoms	Symptoms range from inapparent infection to fulminating and fatal disease, depending on the number of larvae ingested. Symptoms during the initial invasion are nausea, vomiting, diarrhoea and fever. During the phase of parasite dissemination to the tissues, there may be rheumatic manifestations, muscle soreness and pain together with oedema of the upper eyelids, sometimes followed by subconjunctival, subungual and retinal haemorrhages, pain and photophobia. Thirst, profuse sweating, chills, weakness, prostration and rapidly increasing eosinophilia may follow shortly after the ocular symptoms.
Sequelae	Cardiac and neurological complications may appear in weeks 3–6; in the most severe cases death due to myocardial failure may occur.
Duration	2 weeks to 2–3 months.
Reservoir/source	Pigs, dogs, cats, rats, horses and other mammals in the domestic environment.
Mode of transmission and example of foods involved in outbreaks	Ingestion of raw or undercooked meat containing the encysted larvae. Examples of foods involved include pork, horse, game (wild boar, bear).
Specific control measures	*Industrial:* irradiation of meat, freezing, heating and curing. *Food service establishment/household:* thorough cooking of meat, freezing (e.g. minus 15 °C for 30 days). *Consumers:* hunters should thoroughly cook all game.
Occurrence	Worldwide, with predominance in countries where pork or game is eaten.

Type of illness	**Taeniasis:**
	Taenia solium taeniasis and cysticercosis
	Taenia saginata taeniasis
ICD code	ICD-9: 123.0 (*Taenia solium* taeniasis); 123.2 (*Taenia saginata* taeniasis); 123.1 (cysticercosis)
	ICD-10: B68.0 (*Taenia solium* taeniasis); B68.1 (*Taenia saginata* taeniasis); B69 (cysticercosis)
Etiological agent	Helminth (cestode/tapeworm):
	Taenia solium and *Cysticercus cellulosae*[a] (larvae of *T. solium*)
	Taenia saginata and *Cysticercus bovis*[b] (larvae of *T. saginata*).
Characteristics of the agent	*T. solium* causes both intestinal infection with adult worms as well as somatic infection with the eggs. The adult worm comprises a scolex 1 mm in diameter, armed with two rows of hooks and four suckers. The strobila ranges in length from 1.8 m to 4 m. *T. saginata* causes only intestinal infection with adult worms. The adult worm comprises a scolex 1–2 mm in diameter, equipped with four suckers, a neck, and a strobila that ranges in length from 35 mm to 6 m.
Incubation period	Symptoms of cysticercosis appear from a few days to over 10 years. Eggs appear in the stools 8–12 weeks after infection with *T. solium*, and 10–14 weeks after infection with *T. saginata*.
Symptoms	Nervousness, insomnia, anorexia, weight loss, abdominal pain and digestive disturbance. Cysticercosis may cause epileptiform seizures, signs of intracranial hypertension or psychiatric disturbance. Cysticercosis may be fatal.
Sequelae	Cysticercosis may affect the central nervous system. When eggs or proglottides of *T. solium* are swallowed, the eggs hatch in the small intestine and the larvae migrate to subcutaneous tissue, striated muscles, and other tissues and vital organs of the body where they form cysts. Severe health consequences occur when the larvae localize in the eye, central nervous system or heart.
Reservoir/source	Humans; pigs and cattle are the intermediate host for *T. solium* and *T. saginata*.
Mode of transmission and example of foods involved in outbreaks	Taeniasis is caused by consumption of raw or undercooked beef (*Taenia saginata*) or pork (*Taenia solium*) containing cysticerci.
	Gravid proglottides of the parasite are excreted in faeces. Eggs within the

---

[a,b] Names assigned before the organisms were found to be the larval forms of *T. solium* and *T. saginata*, respectively.

	segments are infective. Cattle ingest the eggs deposited on pasture and pigs ingest those deposited on soil. When viable eggs are ingested by cattle or pigs they develop into cysticerci in the muscle. Cysticercosis is caused by ingestion of *T. solium* eggs by the faecal-oral route, person-to-person contact, autoinfection (unwashed hands) or consumption of contaminated food, e.g. vegetables.
Specific control measures	*Industrial:* prevention of faecal contamination of soil, water, human and animal food through safe disposal of sewage; avoidance of sewage water for irrigation use. Irradiation, heat treatment, and freezing kill the cysticerci. *Food service establishment/household:* thorough cooking of meat. *Other:* early diagnosis and treatment to prevent cysticercosis.
Occurrence	Worldwide. Most common in Africa, Latin America, eastern Europe, and south-east Asia. Estimated rate of occurrence varies from + to ++ in high prevalence areas.
Other comments	*T. saginata* eggs are infective only in cattle, *T. solium* eggs are infective in pigs and humans. Eggs of both species are disseminated in the environment as long as the worm remains in the intestine, sometimes for more than 30 years; eggs may remain viable in the environment for months.

Type of illness	Clonorchiasis
ICD code	ICD-9: 121.1 ICD-10: B66.1
Etiological agent	Helminth (trematode/flatworm): *Clonorchis sinensis*, also known as Chinese or oriental liver fluke.
Characteristics of the agent	This is a flattened worm, 10–25 mm long, 3–5 mm wide and usually spatula shaped. It is yellow-brown, owing to bile staining, has an oral and a ventral sucker and is a hermaphrodite. Eggs measure 20–30 μm × 15–17 μm; they are operculate and among the smallest trematode eggs to occur in humans.
Incubation period	Unpredictable: varies with the number of worms present. Symptoms begin with the entry of immature flukes into the biliary system, within one month after encysted larvae (metacercariae) are ingested.
Symptoms	Gradual onset of discomfort in the right upper abdominal quadrant, anorexia, indigestion, abdominal pain or distension and irregular bowel movement. Patients who are heavily infected experience weakness, weight loss, epigastric discomfort, abdominal fullness, diarrhoea, anaemia, oedema. In the later stages, jaundice, portal hypertension, ascites and upper gastointestinal bleeding occur.
Sequelae	The liver (predominantly the left lobe) is enlarged. The spleen can be palpated in only a small percentage of infected cases. Recurrent pyogenic cholangitis is a serious complication of clonorchiasis. The pancreas may be involved in severe cases of *C. sinensis* infection. The pathology of pancreatic clonorchiasis is similar to that of hepatic lesion, namely adenomatous hyperplasia of the ductal epithelium. When acute pancreatitis occurs, features of inflammation are present. Cholangiocarcinoma is also associated with clonorchiasis. Repeated or heavy infection during childhood has been reported to cause dwarfism with retarded sexual development.
Reservoir/source	Snails are the first intermediate host. Some 40 species of river fish serve as the second intermediate host. Humans, dogs, cats and many other species of fish-eating mammals are definitive hosts.
Mode of transmission and example of foods involved in outbreaks	People are infected by eating raw or under-processed freshwater fish containing encysted larvae (metacercariae). During digestion, the larvae are freed from the cysts and migrate via the common bile duct to biliary radicles. Eggs deposited in the bile passages are evacuated in faeces. Eggs in faeces contain fully developed miracidia; when ingested by a susceptible operculate snail, they hatch in its intestine, penetrate the tissues and asexually generate larvae (cercariae) that migrate into the water. On

contact with a second intermediate host, the cercariae penetrate the host and encyst, usually in muscle, occasionally on the underside of scales. The complete life cycle from person to snail to fish to person requires at least 3 months.

Specific control measures	*Industrial*: Safe disposal of excreta and sewage/wastewater to prevent contamination of rivers; treatment of wastewater used for aquaculture; irradiation of freshwater fish; freezing; heat treatment, e.g. canning. *Food service establishment/household*: thorough cooking of freshwater fish. *Consumers* should avoid consumption of raw or undercooked freshwater fish. *Other*: control of snails with molluscicides where feasible; drug treatment of the population to reduce the reservoir of infection; elimination of stray dogs and cats.
Occurrence	Endemic in western Pacific areas: China, Hong Kong SAR, Japan, Malaysia, Republic of Korea, Singapore, Viet Nam. Estimated rate of occurrence: ++/+++. In Europe: east of Russian Federation (estimated rate of occurrence: ++).
Other comments	About one-third of chronic infections are asymptomatic.

Type of illness	Fascioliasis
ICD code	ICD-9: 121.3 ICD-10: B66.3
Etiological agent	Helminth (trematode/flatworm/liver fluke): *Fasciola hepatica* and *Fasciola gigantica*.
Characteristics of the agent	*Fasciola hepatica*: large fluke (23–30 mm × 15 mm), pale grey in colour with dark borders, leaf-shaped with a distinct cephalic cone at the anterior end. Eggs are usually 130–150 µm × 63–90 µm. They have an inconspicuous operculum, are non-embryonated, and often have a shell irregularity at the abopercular end. *Fasciola gigantica* is bigger and may reach a length of 75 mm.
Incubation period	4–6 weeks.
Symptoms	Fever, sweating, abdominal pain, dizziness, cough, bronchial asthma, urticaria. In children, the acute infection is accompanied by severe clinical manifestations, including right upper quadrant pain or generalized abdominal pain, fever and anaemia, and can be fatal. Ectopic infections are common in humans.
Sequelae	Necrotic lesions, inflammatory, adenomatous and fibrotic changes in the bile duct, biliary stasis, atrophy of the liver and periportal cirrhosis, cholecystitis and cholelithiasis.
Reservoir/source	Snails are the intermediate host; sheep, cattle and humans are the definitive hosts.
Mode of transmission and example of foods involved in outbreaks	Infection in humans is associated with the consumption of uncultivated raw watercress (*Nasturtium officinale*) and other salad plants, such as dandelions, bearing metacercariae. After ingestion, the larvae are released from the cyst envelopes into the duodenum, pass through the intestinal wall to the abdominal cavity, enter the liver and after development enter the bile ducts and begin laying non-embryonated eggs 3–4 months after initial exposure. The eggs are carried by the bile into the intestine, and evacuated with the faeces. In suitable temperature and humidity conditions the eggs mature and the miracidia emerge from the eggs into the water in a few weeks. The miracidia penetrate the snail (intermediate host), turn into sporocysts and in about 3 weeks produce rediae which, in turn, produce cercariae. The cercariae may begin to emerge from the snails in 6 weeks under favourable conditions. After leaving the snail, the cercariae swim in the water and encyst on vegetation, turning into metacercariae which can survive for a long time in a wet environment. The life cycle is then complete.

Specific control measures	*Industrial*: Safe disposal of excreta and sewage/wastewater; drug treatment of livestock against the parasite; prevention of animal access to commercial watercress beds and control of water used to irrigate the beds. *Food service establishment/household*: thorough cooking of food. *Consumers* should avoid consumption of raw watercress. *Other*: control of snails with molluscicides where feasible; drug treatment of the population to reduce the reservoir of infection.
Occurrence	Africa, e.g. Egypt, Ethiopia; Americas, e.g. Bolivia, Ecuador, Peru; Asia, e.g. Islamic Republic of Iran; Europe: France, Portugal, Spain; and the western Pacific, e.g. China. The estimated rate of occurrence varies, depending on the country, from ++ to +++.

Type of illness	Opisthorchiasis
ICD code	ICD-9: 121.0 ICD-10: B66.0
Etiological agent	Helminth (trematode/flatworm/liver fluke): *Opisthorchis viverrini* and *Opisthorchis felineus.*
Characteristics of the agent	Morphological features ressemble those of *Clonorchis sinensis.* The worm lives in the intrahepatic bile ducts and pancreas and has been also found in the lungs. It measures 8–11 mm × 1.5–2 mm. Eggs measure 30 μm × 12 μm and are slenderer than the *C. sinensis* eggs.
Incubation period	2–4 weeks, very occasionally 1 week.
Symptoms	Fever, abdominal pain, dizziness, urticaria. Chronic cases may lead to diarrhoea, flatulence, fatty food intolerance, epigastric and right upper quadrant pain, jaundice, fever, hepatomegaly, lassitude, anorexia, and in some cases emaciation and oedema.
Sequelae	Cholecystitis, cholangitis, liver abscess and gallstones. Cholangiocarcinoma is associated with *O. viverrini* infection and perhaps also with *O. felineus.*
Reservoir/source	The first intermediate host is the freshwater snail; several fish species act as second intermediate host. Humans, dogs, cats, and other mammals that eat fish or fish waste are definitive hosts.
Mode of transmission and example of foods involved in outbreaks	Humans are infected by consumption of raw or under-processed freshwater fish. The life cycle of *Opisthorchis* spp. is similar to that of *C. sinesis.*
Specific control measures	*Industrial*: Safe disposal of excreta and sewage/wastewater; treatment of wastewater used for aquaculture; irradiation of freshwater fish; freezing; heat treatment, e.g. canning. *Food service establishment/household*: thorough cooking of freshwater fish. Consumers should avoid consumption of raw or undercooked freshwater fish. *Other*: control of snails with molluscicides where feasible; drug treatment of the population to reduce the reservoir of infection; elimination of stray dogs and cats.
Occurrence	*Opisthorchis viverrini*: Cambodia, Lao People's Democratic Republic, Thailand.

Opisthorchis felineus: Europe: Baltic states, eastern Germany, Kazakhstan, Poland, the Russian Federation, Ukraine; Asia: India, Japan, Thailand. The estimated rate of occurrence is ++ in European countries and +++ in Asian countries.

Type of illness	Paragonimiasis
ICD code	ICD-9: 121.2 ICD-10: B66.4
Etiological agent	Helminth (trematode/flatworm/lung fluke): *Paragonimus westermani* (metacercariae).
Characteristics of the agent	This is a reddish brown hermaphrodite which measures 10–12 mm in length and 5–7 mm in width (adult). The shape varies from linear to spherical. Eggs usually measure 80–120 µm, are golden brown in colour, thick-shelled, non-embryonated in faeces or in sputum and have a prominent operculum. The shell is thickened at the abopercular end.
Incubation period	Acute stage: a few days to several weeks. Chronic stage: pulmonary symptoms begin at around 3 months.
Symptoms	The early stages are usually asymptomatic. However, heavily infected patients may experience fever, fatigue, generalized myalgia and abdominal pain with eosinophilia.
Sequelae	Pleuropulmonary paragonimiasis (pulmonary lesion): chronic coughing, thoracic pain, blood-stained viscous sputum. Systemic symptoms of fatigue, fever, myalgia, chest pain and dyspnoea. Severe infections produce tuberculosis-like symptoms. Ectopic paragonimiasis (extrapulmonary lesion): migration of the worm through the brain can cause cerebral haemorrhage, oedema or meningitis. Severe headache, mental confusion, seizure, hemiparesis, hypaesthesia, blurred vision, diplopia, homonymous hemianopsia and meningismus may occur. Abdominal paragonimiasis: results in abdominal pain, and there may be diarrhoea with blood and mucus when the intestinal mucosa is ulcerated.
Reservoir/source	Freshwater snails are the first intermediate host; crabs and crayfish are second intermediate hosts. Humans, dogs, pigs and other wild and domestic animals are definitive hosts.
Mode of transmission and example of foods involved in outbreaks	The definitive hosts are infected through consumption of raw, inadequately cooked or otherwise under-processed freshwater crustaceans (crabs and crayfish) which contain the metacercariae, or through contamination of other food items, hands and cooking utensils by the metacercariae released from infected crabs during food preparation. Following ingestion the metacercariae in the infected crustaceans excyst in the duodenum of the host and the larvae penetrate the intestinal wall and migrate beneath the peritoneum where they remain for 5–7 days. Over a period of about 2–3 weeks following infection, the immature worms penetrate the

diaphragm, enter the pleural cavity and then move into the lung parenchyma where they mature. At this stage, eggs may be present in the sputum without the host showing any symptoms. During the initial stage of lung infection, the adult worms migrate through the tissues and cause focal haemorrhagic pneumonia. After 12 weeks, the worms in the lung parenchyma typically provoke a granulomatous reaction that gradually proceeds to development of fibrotic encapsulation. Extrapulmonary lesions are caused by worms that reach and develop in ectopic foci.

Specific control measures	*Industrial*: safe disposal of excreta and sewage/wastewater to prevent contamination of rivers.
	Food service establishment/household: thorough cooking of crabs and crayfish, and hygienic handling of these foods.
	Consumers should avoid consumption of raw or undercooked or under-processed crabs and crayfish.
	Other: control of snails with molluscicides where feasible; drug treatment of the population to reduce the reservoir of infection; elimination of stray dogs and cats.
Occurrence	Africa, e.g. Cameroon, Nigeria; Americas, e.g. Ecuador, Peru; Asia, e.g. China, Japan, Lao People's Democratic Republic, Philippines, Republic of Korea, Thailand. Estimated rate of occurrence in these countries is $+++$.

Bibliography

Benenson AS, ed. *Control of communicable diseases manual: an official report of the American Public Health Association*, 16th ed. Washington, DC, American Public Health Association, 1995.

Foodborne pathogens: risk and consequences. Taskforce report. Ames, IA, USA Council of Agricultural Science and Technology, 1994.

Hobbs B, Roberts D. *Food poisoning and food hygiene*, 6th ed. London, Edward Arnold, 1993.

Management of outbreaks of foodborne illness. London, Department of Health, 1994.

Motarjemi Y, Käferstein FK. Global estimation of foodborne diseases. *World health statistics quarterly*, 1997, 50(1/2):5–11.

Quevedo F, Thakur AS. *Foodborne parasitic diseases.* Washington, DC, Pan American Health Organization, 1990 (Series of scientific and technical monographs Number 12, Rev. 1).

Risk communication[1]

Definition and goals

Risk communication is the exchange of information and opinions concerning risk and risk-related factors among risk assessors, risk managers, consumers and other interested parties. The fundamental goal of risk communication is to provide meaningful, relevant and accurate information, in clear and understandable terms targeted to a specific audience.

The goals of risk communication are:

— to promote awareness and understanding of the specific issues under consideration during the risk analysis process, by all participants;

— to promote consistency and transparency in arriving at and implementing risk management[2] decisions;

— to provide a sound basis for understanding the risk management decisions proposed or implemented;

— to improve the overall effectiveness and efficiency of the risk analysis process;

— to contribute to the development and delivery of effective information and education programmes, when they are selected as risk management options;

— to foster public trust and confidence in the safety of the food supply;

— to strengthen working relationships and mutual respect among all participants;

— to promote the appropriate involvement of all interested parties in the risk communication process;

— to exchange information on the knowledge, attitudes, values, practices and perceptions of interested parties concerning risks associated with food and related topics.

---

[1] Excerpted from: *The application of risk communication to food standards and safety matters. The Report of a Joint FAO/WHO Expert Consultation, Rome, 2-6 February 1998.* Rome, Food and Agriculture Organization of the United Nations, 1999 (FAO Food and Nutrition Paper, No. 70).

[2] Risk management is the process of weighing policy alternatives in the light of the results of risk assessment and, if required, selecting and implementing appropriate control options, including regulatory measures.

Elements of risk communication

Depending on what is to be communicated and to whom, risk communication messages may contain information on the following:

The nature of the risk

- The characteristics and importance of the hazard of concern.
- The magnitude and severity of the risk.
- The urgency of the situation.
- Whether the risk is becoming greater or smaller (trends).
- The probability of exposure to the hazard.
- The distribution of exposure.
- The amount of exposure that constitutes a significant risk.
- The nature and size of the population at risk.
- Who is at the greatest risk.

The nature of the benefits

- The actual or expected benefits associated with each risk.
- Who benefits and in what ways.
- Where the balance point is between risks and benefits.
- The magnitude and importance of the benefits.
- The total benefit to all affected populations combined.
- Uncertainties in risk assessment.
- The methods used to assess the risk.
- The importance of each of the uncertainties.
- The weaknesses of, or inaccuracies in, the available data.
- The assumptions on which estimates are based.
- The sensitivity of the estimates to changes in assumptions.
- The effect of changes in the estimates on risk management decisions.

Risk management options

- The action(s) taken to control or manage the risk.
- The action individuals may take to reduce personal risk.
- The justification for choosing a specific risk management option.
- The effectiveness of a specific option.
- The benefits of a specific option.
- The cost of managing the risk, and who pays for it.
- The risks that remain after a risk management option is implemented.

Principles of risk communication

Know the audience

In formulating risk communication messages, the audience should be analysed in order to understand their motivations and opinions. Beyond knowing in general who the audience is, it is necessary to get to know them as groups and ideally as individuals to understand their concerns and feelings and to maintain an open channel of communication with them. Listening to all interested parties is an important part of risk communication.

Involve the scientific experts

Scientific experts, in their capacity as risk assessors, must be able to explain the concepts and processes of risk assessment. They need to be able to explain the results of their assessment and the scientific data, assumptions and subjective judgements upon which it is based, so that risk managers and other interested parties clearly understand the risk. They must be able to communicate clearly what they know and what they do not know, and to explain the uncertainties related to the risk assessment process. In turn, risk managers must be able to explain how risk management decisions are arrived at.

Establish expertise in communication

Successful risk communication requires expertise in conveying understandable and usable information to all interested parties. Risk managers and technical experts may not have the time or skill to perform complex risk communication tasks, such as responding to the needs of various audiences (public, industry, media etc.) and preparing effective messages. People with expertise in risk communication should therefore be involved as early as possible. This expertise will probably have to be developed by training and experience.

Be a credible source of information

Information from credible sources is more likely to influence the public perception of a risk than is information from sources that lack this attribute. The credibility accorded a source by a target audience may vary according to the nature of the hazard, culture, social and economic status, and other factors. If consistent messages are received from multiple sources, the credibility of the message is reinforced. Factors determining credibility of the source include recognized competence or expertise, trustworthiness, fairness, and lack of bias. For example, the terms that consumers have associated with high credibility include "factual", "knowledgeable", "expert", "public welfare", "responsible", "truthful", and "good track record". Trust and credibility must be nurtured and can be eroded or lost through ineffective or inappropriate communication. In studies, consumers have indicated that distrust and low credibility result from exaggeration, distortion and perceived vested interest.

Effective communications acknowledge current issues and problems, are open in their content and approach, and are timely. Timeliness of the message is most important since many controversies become focused on the question "why didn't you tell us sooner?" rather than on the risk itself. Omissions, distortions and self-serving statements will damage credibility in the longer term.

Share responsibility

Regulatory agencies of governments at national, regional and local levels have a fundamental responsibility for risk communication. The public expects the government to play a leading role in managing public health risks. This is true when the risk management decision involves regulatory or voluntary controls, and is even true when the government decision is to take no action. In the latter event, communication is still essential to provide reasons why taking no action is the best option. In order to understand the public concerns and to ensure that risk management decisions respond to those concerns in appropriate ways, the government needs to determine what the public knows about the risks and what the public thinks of the various options being considered to manage those risks.

The media play an essential role in the communication process and therefore share in these responsibilities. Communication on immediate risks involving human health, particularly when there is a potential for serious health consequences such as in the case of foodborne illnesses, cannot be treated in the same way as less immediate food safety concerns. Industry also has a responsibility for risk communication, especially when the risk is a result of its products or processes. All parties in the risk communication process (e.g. government, industry, media) have joint responsibility for the outcome even though their individual roles may differ. Since science must be the basis for decision-making, all parties in the communication process should know the basic principles and data supporting the risk assessment and the policies underlying the risk management decisions.

Differentiate between science and value judgement

It is essential to separate facts from values in considering risk management options. At a practical level, it is useful to report the facts that are known at the time as well as what uncertainties are involved in the risk management decisions being proposed or implemented. The risk communicator has the responsibility to explain what is known as fact and where the limits of this knowledge begin and end. Value judgements are involved in the concept of acceptable levels of risk. Consequently, risk communicators should be able to justify the level of acceptable risk to the public. Many people take the term "safe food" to mean food with zero risk, but zero risk is often unattainable. In practice, "safe food" usually means food that is safe enough. Making this clear is an important function of risk communication.

Assure transparency

If the public are to accept the risk analysis process and its outcomes, the process must be transparent. While respecting legitimate concerns to preserve confidentiality (e.g. proprietary information or data), transparency in risk analysis consists of having the process open and available for scrutiny by interested parties. Effective two-way communication between risk managers, the public and interested parties is both an essential part of risk management and a key to achieving transparency.

Put the risk in perspective

One way to put a risk in perspective is to examine it in the context of the benefits associated with the technology or process that poses the risk. Another approach that may be helpful is to compare the risk at issue with other similar, more familiar risks. However, this latter approach can create problems if it appears that risk comparisons have been intentionally chosen to make the risk at issue seem more acceptable to the public. In general, risk comparisons should not be used unless:

— both (or all) risk estimates are equally sound;
— both (or all) risk estimates are relevant to the specific audience;
— the degree of uncertainty in all risk estimates is similar;
— the concerns of the audience are acknowledged and addressed;
— the substances, products or activities themselves are directly comparable, including the concept of voluntary and involuntary exposure.

General requirements for effective risk communication

Many considerations for effective risk communication, especially those involving the public, can be grouped in a sequence following the systematic approach of the risk communication process. This starts with gathering background and needed information, followed by the preparation and assembly of the message, its dissemination and distribution, and a follow-up review and evaluation of its impact.

Background and information

- Understand the scientific basis of the risks and attendant uncertainties.
- Understand the public perception of the risk through such means as risk surveys, interviews and focus groups.
- Find out what risk information people want.
- Be sensitive to related issues that may be more important to people than the risk itself.
- Expect different people to see the risk differently.

Preparation and assembly

- Avoid comparisons between familiar risks and new risks, as they may seem flippant and insincere unless presented properly.
- Recognize and respond to the emotional aspects of risk perceptions. Speak with sympathy and never use logic alone to convince an audience characterized by emotion.
- Express risk in several different ways, making sure not to evade the risk question.
- Explain the uncertainty factors which are used in risk assessment and standard setting.
- Maintain an openness, flexibility, and recognition of public responsibilities in all communication activities.
- Build an awareness of benefits associated with a risk.

Dissemination/distribution

- Accept and involve the public as a legitimate partner by describing risk/benefit information and control measures in an understandable way.
- Share the public's concern rather than deny it as not legitimate or as unimportant. Be prepared to give people's concerns as much emphasis as the risk statistics.
- Be honest, frank, and open in discussing all issues.
- If explaining statistics derived from risk assessment, explain the risk assessment process before presenting the numbers.
- Coordinate and collaborate with other credible sources.
- Meet the needs of the media.

Review/evaluation

- Evaluate the effectiveness of risk messages and communication channels.
- Emphasize action to monitor, manage, and reduce risk.
- Plan carefully and evaluate efforts.

Points to consider regarding public concerns

Risks that involve some or all of the following aspects tend to concern the public more than those risks that lack these aspects:

— unknown, unfamiliar or rare events as opposed to well-known or common hazards;

— risks controlled by others, rather than those where the public or the individual is in control;

— risks that result from the action of industry or new technology, rather than those perceived as natural;

— risks where there is significant scientific uncertainty, or where there is open controversy among experts as to the probability and severity of the hazard;

— risks that raise moral or ethical questions, such as the fairness of the distribution of risks and benefits, or the rights of one group in society to put others at risk;

— the decision-making process by which the risk is assessed is seen as being unresponsive or is unknown.

Therefore, in order to mitigate public concern about risks, the following strategies may be used:

- Make risks voluntary by giving consumers choices, whenever possible.
- Acknowledge uncertainty.
- Show that expert disagreement on an issue is merely uncertainty, by estimating risks as a range that includes estimates from both sides of the debate.
- Determine where control is and look to share it with interested parties.
- Treat all interested parties with courtesy.
- Always consider concerns and complaints seriously.